*Nature's Cures for
Degenerative Health Problems:*
*Heart Disease, Diabetes, Cancer, Arthritis,
Allergies, Aging, etc.*

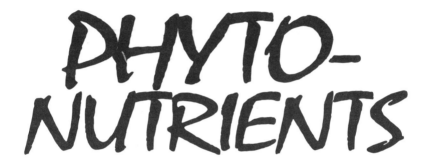
PHYTO-NUTRIENTS

MEDICINAL NUTRIENTS FOUND IN FOOD
REVISED AND UPDATED

**A Health Learning Handbook
Beth M. Ley, Ph.D.**

BL Publications
Detroit Lakes, MN

Copyright © 1998, 2007 (Updated)
No part of this publication may be reproduced, stored in a retrieval system or transmitted in any form by any means, electronic, mechanical, photocopy, recording or otherwise, without the prior permission of the publisher, except as provided by USA copyright law.

ISBN: 0-9642703-9-0

All rights reserved. No part of this book may be reproduced or transmitted by any means, electronic or mechanical, without written permission from the publisher:

BL Publications
Detroit Lakes, MN 56501
877- BOOKS11
www.blpublications.com
Sign up for our FREE monthly newsletter!

Printed in the United States of America

This book is not intended as medical advice. Its purpose is solely educational. Please consult your healthcare professional for all health problems.

Cover design: BL Publications/ Jeritta Gronewold

YOU NEED TO KNOW...
THE HEALTH MESSAGE

Do you not know that you are God's temple and that God's Spirit dwells in you? If anyone destroys God's temple, God will destroy him, For God's temple is holy and that temple you are. *1 Cor. 3:16-17*

So, whether you eat or drink, or whatever you do, do all to the glory of God. *1 Cor. 10:31*

TABLE OF CONTENTS

Introduction 4

Phytonutrients Defined 5

Free Radicals and Free Radical Diseases 7

Antioxidants 10

ORAC: Measuring Antioxidant Power 11

Important Antioxidant-Rich Foods: 16

My Healthiest Foods List 23
    Vegetables 23
    Fruits 36
    Beans & Legumes 47
    Nuts & Seeds 49
    Grains 52
    Spices & Herbs 55

Phytochemical/Food Chart 60-61

Bibliography .62-63

Other Books from BL Publications 64

Introduction

Good health should not be thought of as the absence of disease. We should avoid this negative disease-orientated thinking and concentrate on what we must to do to remain healthy. Health results from supplying what is essential to the body on a daily basis, while disease results from living without what the body needs. We are responsible for our own health and should take control of it before diseases does.

Our health depends on education. Education is power.

I like to call this book "all the cool stuff God put in our food to make us healthy!" There are hundreds and hundreds of chemicals identified in our foods that have amazing health promoting properties. If we would only eat the foods that God made (instead of man-made and processed foods where these valuable components are removed), I am convinced so many people wouldn't be sick, overweight, constipated and taking the tons of pharmaceuticals drugs that people do everyday.

So much new research has come out in the last ten years since I originally came out with this book that the new edition is almost double the size of the original, but I feel that once you read all the benefits of God's foods you will be inspired to change your diet!

Epidemiological studies indicate that a diet rich in fruits and vegetables may lower the incidence of cancer and other degenerative conditions. This preventive effect of fruits and vegetables could be due to the numerous benefits that these foods provide us with. They are low in calories, low in fat, and provide us with various vitamins, minerals, antioxidants and **phytochemicals** - specific medicinal compounds derived from plants. (Hocman)

> *Every bite of fruit or vegetable contains thousands of phytochemicals which promote and protect our health!*

PhytoNutrients Defined

"Phyto" is derived from the Greek word for plants. Phytonutrients include the pigment chemicals which give plants their colors (green, yellow, blue, purple, red, orange), fatty molecules like sterols and essential fatty acids, vitamins and minerals, plus more complicated chemicals called polysaccharides. There are literally thousands of these chemicals (many, if not most of them, not even identified yet) which can provide various health benefits, such as supporting healthy brain, organ, and immune function, plus promote healthy circulation and hormone balance.

Phytochemicals are designed to protect the plant from sunlight or certain pathogens (like an immune system for the plant itself), but also offers protection for those who eat the plant. Phytochemicals have biochemical properties which go far beyond vitamins, minerals and even antioxidant nutrients in their ability to protect us from the multiple processes that lead to cancer and other health problems.

In a thorough review headed by Gladys Block, M.D., at the National Cancer Institute, Bethesda, MD, the inverse relationship between fruit and vegetable intake and many types of common cancer was clearly demonstrated. They specifically noted studies on cancer such as lung, colon, breast, cervix, and esophagus. (Patterson)

Researchers are discovering how many of the hundreds (if not thousands) of different phytonutrients in fruits and vegetables enhance the immune system and prevent disease. The mechanisms of prevention include enhanced enzymatic detoxification of harmful compounds, and inhibition of their binding to cellular DNA, their fiber content, detoxification of radical forms of carcinogens by their natural antioxidants and probably many other ways too.

Free radicals play a critical role in the development of the two diseases responsible for 2 out of every 3 deaths. The Mayo Clinic reports that approximately 43% of deaths in the United States are due to some form of cardiovascular disease, and 23% are caused by cancer.

Almost 10 years ago the Surgeon Generals Report on Nutrition and Health stated that making the correct dietary choices could decrease our cancer risk by 35 to 60%. The National Cancer Institute (NCI) even opened a Cancer Research Laboratory devoted solely to investigating the role of diet in cancer prevention and treatment. Numerous studies have already demonstrated the protective relationship between fruit and vegetable intake and cancers of the lung, colon, breast, cervix, esophagus, mouth and throat, stomach, bladder, pancreas, and ovary.

While the U.S. Surgeon General recommends 5-9 servings of fruits and vegetables daily, the *Journal of Nutrition* reports that just one out of 10 Americans eats this amount. We are to eat them raw or cooked, preferably lightly steamed and not microwaved which can destroy their delicate balance of anticarcinogenic ingredients. Recent studies show microwaving broccoli destroys up to 97% of certain flavonoids.

The September 2006 *Journal of the American Dietetic Association* reported that less than 40% of Americans consume at least five servings of fruits and vegetables per day. Dark green and orange vegetables and legumes were the most lacking from people's diets, with current intakes less than a third of the recommended amounts.

Why don't we eat our fruits and veggies?

1. It's difficult to get to the market everyday to purchase a fresh supply.

2. Time required for preparation.

3. Expense.

4. Pesticides and other chemicals contaminate our produce making it extremely difficult to find 100% pure fruits and vegetables.

5. And finally, not everyone likes the taste of certain foods.

> Most people like fruit, but how many of us actually eat the 5-9 servings recommended by the U.S. Surgeon General?
>
> Only one in five persons according to a phone survey published in The *American Journal of Public Health* in 1995. (Surdula) Other reports say one in 10!

Free Radicals & Free Radical Diseases

Researchers around the world tell us that free radical damage throughout the body is a major cause of aging and age-associated diseases.

A free radical is an incomplete, unstable molecule. It is incomplete because it is missing an electron which exists in pairs in stable molecules. It is unstable because it will "steal" an electron from another molecule, and thereby create another free radical and a chain reaction of events, which results in thousands of reactions.

Every time molecules lose or gain an electron, they are weakened and, ultimately, the whole structure, whether it is an enzyme, a protein, a cell membrane, tissues, or even organs, is damaged. Some areas of the body are more susceptible to damage than others.

Free radicals can attack and damage cells from the inside or outside of the cell. The main targets for free radical attack are the vulnerable lipid-composed membranes of cells and their inner structures: the mitochondria, the Golgi functions and the endoplasmic reticulum, the nuclear membrane, etc. Damage to genetic material (DNA and RNA) is associated with cell abnormalities and cancer.

Free radicals damage fatty compounds circulating in the blood stream, causing damage and the release of more free radicals in a chain reaction. Damage to LDL and

Lipoprotein(a) are associated with heart disease.

Free radicals destroy protein as seen in cataract formation, kidney damage, and damage to hemoglobin cells and aging in general (collagen breakdown).

Free radicals create cross-linking. When free radicals damage molecules, cells split off to repair the injury. The cells have to rejoin with others to reform and reshape themselves. This may cause cross linkage, a bond between large amino acid molecules which are normally separate from each other. Additional free radicals are also formed when waste fragments of these molecules break off. Many people realize that cross-linkages cause wrinkles, but they also cause "aging" throughout the entire body. Free radicals cause proteins (i.e., collagen tissue) and/or genetic material (i.e., DNA) to fuse. Healthy DNA is necessary to replicate and renew the body's cellular components. Altered DNA produces useless debris and sometimes cancerous cells.

Free radical reactions form age pigments (residues called lipofuscin). These residues accumulate with time and interfere with cell function and life processes.

When free radicals destroy cell membranes, they are interfering with the cell's ability to absorb nutrients and expel waste products. Without this ability, the cell dies. Cell membrane damage can lead to numerous degenerative problems and accelerated aging.

Production of free radicals is a normal part of the body's mechanism. There are tens of thousands of free radicals formed in the body every second. However, they are not all harmful; some actually help us. The body's immune system uses free radicals to kill potentially infectious microbes and viruses. This activity (called phagocytosis), however, at the same time creates even more free radicals (hydrogen peroxide and hydroxyl radicals) that may lead to severe tissue damage.

Our daily exposure to environmental free radicals is a major contributor to the level of free radicals in the body.

Free radicals are major factors in about 80 different diseases, including: (Ames)

Heart disease and stroke	**Cancer (all types)**
Diabetes (esp. type 2)	**Cataracts**
Macular degeneration	**Allergies**
Arthritis and Lupus	**Asthma**
Pancreatitis	**Neuropathy**
Inflammatory bowel disease	**Aging**
Other inflammatory conditions	
Alzheimer's and other neuro-degenerative diseases	
Other neurological diseases	

Some external sources of free radicals are:
- Cigarette smoke
- Environmental pollutants (smog, etc.)
- Radiation
- Ultraviolet light
- Certain drugs, pesticides, anaesthetics and industrial solvents
- Ozone

Other factors which increase your need for antioxidants include: **Exercise; Stress; Illness, infection, inflammation**, and many health problems - diabetes, arthritis, asthma; **Elevated blood lipids** (especially LDL); **Elevated blood sugar**, Many stimulants and metabolic enhancers such as caffeine and diet pills;

Free Radicals Accelerate Aging. Aging also results from the loss of vital cells from free radical reactions. Free radicals destroy the membranes of lysosomes, enzyme-containing organelles found inside most cells. If the membrane sac that stores these enzymes is ruptured, the enzymes will kill the cell. With each cell destroyed and without the ability to renew itself, we become one cell older.

Antioxidants

Compounds which prevent the process of free radical degeneration are called **antioxidants.** Antioxidants are a class of nutrients which possess the ability to destroy free radicals and thus prevent the diseases associated with free radical damage. Antioxidants also help alleviate the symptoms and side-effects of many of these diseases.

Low levels of antioxidants increase free radical activity and are clearly associated with an increased risk of health problems. Therefore, the use of antioxidant supplements to scavenge free radicals can potentially decrease the risks of cancer, cardiovascular disease, cataracts, macular degeneration, neuropathy and other circulatory problems and the many other degenerative conditions. (Barber)

Free radicals damage cells and tissues throughout the body. These radicals act on different structures, and the use of various antioxidants exert various favorable effects. Our genetics may make us sensitive to certain health problems such as heart disease or diabetes, but location of the free radical exposure or formation also plays a significant role in the type of damage which results. For example, UV exposure is damaging to the skin and the eyes, and elevated LDL cholesterol molecules circulating in our veins are more susceptible to damage causing arterial plaque to buildup. Smoking damages the throat and lungs, etc.

As long as the ratio of oxidants to antioxidants remains in balance, the negative effects of the free radicals can be controlled. When the balance becomes upset by excessive exposure to internal or external factors or a combination of both, the antioxidants produced by the body simply cannot cope with the increased amount of free radicals.

Diet Alone is Inadequate!

Some lifestyle factors increase your need for special protection offered through phytonutrients. And diet alone does not always provide adequate amounts. Taking large

> Do you not know that you are God's temple and that God's Spirit dwells in you? If any one destroys God's temple, God will destroy him, For God's temple is holy and that temple you are. *I Corinthians 3:16-17*
>
> **How important it is to eat the foods God made for us to eat... Just look at the result (the list of health problems above) of NOT doing so! These conditions are all known to be preventable through a proper diet rich in fruits, vegetables, fiber and whole grains.**

amounts of only one type of phytonutrient, such as beta-carotene, may impair absorption of other carotenes and important nutrients so it is very important to get a **wide variety** of these important nutrients.

The U.S. Department of Health and the NCI recommend that our daily diets provide a minimum of 5 to 6 mg. of just carotenoids (not to mention all other just-as-important phytonutrients). Most diets only provide 1.5 mg.

Strength in Numbers!

There are many different types of free radicals and therefore we require many different types of antioxidants and phytochemicals from a variety of sources to effectively fight off free radical damage.

ORAC: Measuring Antioxidant Power

ORAC (Oxygen Radical Absorbance Capacity) is a test tube analysis that measures the total antioxidant power of foods and other chemical substances. Early findings suggest that eating plenty of high-ORAC fruits and vegetables, such as spinach and blueberries, may help slow the processes associated with aging in both body and brain.

Top-Scoring Fruits & Vegetables
ORAC units per 100 grams (about 3 1/2 oz.)

Fruits	Vegetables
Prunes 5,770	Kale 1,770
Raisins 2,830	Spinach 1,260
Blueberries 2,400	Brussels sprouts 980
Blackberries 2,036	Alfalfa sprouts 930
Strawberries 1,540	Broccoli flowers 890
Raspberries 1,220	Beets 840
Plums 949	Red bell pepper 710
Oranges 750	Onion 450
Red grapes 739	Corn 400
Cherries 670	Eggplant 390
Kiwi fruit 602	
Grapefruit, pink 483	

Scientific contact: Ronald Prior, James Joseph, Guohua Cao or Barbara Shukitt-Hale, Jean Mayer USDA Human Nutrition Research Center on Aging at Tufts, Boston, Mass., phone (617) 557-3310,

3,000 to 5,000 ORAC units per day are suggested by the researchers at the USDA to promote optimal levels in the blood and tissues. However, studies show that the average person gets only about 1,200 ORAC units per day from 3 servings of fruits and vegetables. Supplements can pack a much greater punch gram for gram.

The USDA and other health authorities also stress getting all of the colors in your diet on a regular basis. Interestingly, each color group seems to provide targeted protection to specific areas of the body. For example:

Blue: *Protects the Brain*

Green: *Strengthens the Immune System (detox)*

Yellow: *Protects the Eyes and Blood Pressure*

Orange: *Supports Heart Health*

Red: *Wards off Cancer*

Antioxidants In Our Food:

Vitamin C (ascorbic acid), as an antioxidant, is very effective against free radicals. Vitamin C also stimulates white blood cells and overall immune function. It is effective against hydroxyl and superoxide radicals. Vitamin C also stimulates white blood cells and overall immune function. Vitamin C is found in citrus fruits and some green vegetables, but supplementation is usually required to obtain therapeutic effects.

If you are going to supplement Vitamin C in amounts over 500 mg. per day (which I do recommend), I strongly suggest taking a buffered form such as calcium ascorbate or mineral ascorbate (like is found in fruits) which will not interfere with the pH of the body.

Vitamin E (a-tocopherol) is a major fat-soluble membrane antioxidant found in cells which fights off damage from peroxyl radicals. Vitamin E also protects white blood cells and may retard the decline of immunity which accompanies aging.

Carotenoid complexes are found in colored fruits such an cantaloupe and papaya, and vegetables such as carrots, tomatoes and red grapes. Carotenoids are antioxidants which protect our genetic material from free radical attack. It also suppresses the gene (N-myc) that promotes tumor growth. This gene is part of healthy and nature cells, but is dormant unless damaged by free radicals or switched on by faulty biochemical signals. Cells treated with carotenoids show 24% lower N-myc activity than untreated cells. Even 18 hours later, the activity was 18% lower. (Okuzumi)

Carotenoids also increase our number of white blood cells strengthening our immune system.

Beta-Carotene is one of the best known carotenoids. It is found in fruits such as cantaloupe and peaches and vegetables such as carrots, broccoli, celery, greens, kale, leeks, parsley, spinach, and tomatoes. Algae is also an excellent source of beta-carotene as well as other carotenoids.

Other carotenoids include the following:

Alpha-carotene (carrots, beet greens, yellow peppers, pumpkin, algae)

Cryptoxanthin (papaya, tangerines)

Lutein and **Zeaxanthin** (spinach, tomatoes, kale, parsley, celery, leeks, pumpkin, yellow, green and red peppers, swiss chard). These two carotenoids are recognized for their ability to protect us against macular degeneration and also lung and breast cancer.

Lycopenes (red grapefruit, tomatoes, apricots, scallions, watermelon) Lycopene has specifically drawn attention lately because of its ability to protect us from cancer, especially prostate, skin and pancreatic. While there are over 500 carotenoids found in plants, lycopene is the most abundant carotenoids in human blood and tissues, with levels far above those of beta carotene. Lycopene is a much more potent antioxidant than beta carotene and thus better able to protect us from free radical damage.

Lycopene is what makes tomatoes red and accounts for 70% of the carotenoids in ripe tomatoes. The darker red the tomato, the higher the lycopene content. The only other common foods containing lycopene are grapefruit and watermelon.

Lycopene is fat soluble so it requires a small amount of fat to be consumed with it in order for it to be absorbed into the blood stream. This means that just drinking plain tomato juice won't do you much good in regards to the lycopene it contains. But, the lycopene in spaghetti sauce which contains a small amount of olive oil, is highly absorbable.

Bioflavonoids are members of the flavonol family of compounds and are semi-essential, secondary food factors. There are over 20,000 different registered bioflavonoids found in **fruits and vegetables**, especially **citrus** and **berries**, and various other plants.

Research shows that **flavonoids** keep cancer-causing hormones from latching onto cells. Flavonoids are effective vitamin C potentiators, enabling it to work better and longer in our bodies.

Curcumin (from turmeric), widely used as a spice and coloring agent in food, belongs to the flavonoid family and possesses potent antioxidant, anti-inflammatory, anti-tumor and anti-viral promoting activities. Curcuminoids can also reduce cholesterol levels by almost 30%.

Proanthocyanidins are a group of especially potent bioflavonoids.

Alpha Lipoic Acid, also known as thiotic acid, has several unique properties. Alpha Lipoic Acid is both fat and water soluble, meaning it can protect inside and outside of our cellular membranes.

Lipoic acid also has regenerative properties for other antioxidants such as C, E, and glutathione. Instead of getting "used up" after donating an electron, lipoic acid can recycle them by offering these antioxidants an electron.

Lipoic acid demonstrates powerful therapeutic properties for diabetes and is used throughout Europe to treat and prevent polyneuropathy, cataracts and macular degeneration.

Lipoic acid is naturally found in foods such as potatoes, carrots and yams.

Co-Enzyme Q10 (CoQ10) is an important antioxidant nutrient necessary for intracellular mitochondrial energy production. CoQ10 is depleted through age, disease or inadequate nutrition. As levels decline, immune deficiency opens the door for many disease states. Certain organs of the body require larger concentrations of Co-Q10, such as the heart and liver. CoQ10 as a supplement has proven to reduce blood pressure, stimulate the immune system and improve energy.

All tissues in man contain COQ10. It is found in concentrated amounts inside the cells, especially the mitochondria, which are responsible for producing more than 90% of the energy from our cells. CoQ10 facilitates electron transfer for the production of ATP (usable energy). CoQ10 is utilized in the metabolism of carbohydrates and fats for the production of ATP.

Because the heart muscle has the highest concentration of CoQ10, one can logically assume that it plays an important role in heart health, and it does!

The benefits of CoQ10 to the heart and cardiovascular system have been extensively documented. As an antioxidant, CoQ10 protects low-density lipoprotein (LDL) cholesterol from oxidation (Thomas), and reduces the negative effects of stress by protecting and stabilizing mitochondrial membranes.

Clinical trials have already investigated the relationship between CoQ10 and blood pressure, total LDL and high-density lipoprotein (HDL) cholesterol (Digiesi) and blood platelets which determine our clotting risk potential.

Important Antioxidant-Rich Foods

Acai Berries

Acai (ah-SAH'-ee) berries are considered one of the richest fruit sources of antioxidants. This dark purple Brazilian berry (about the size and shape of a blueberry) contains antioxidants that destroyed cultured human cancer cells in a recent University of Florida study. Published in the *Journal of Agricultural and Food Chemistry (January 2006)*, the study showed extracts from acai berries triggered a self-destruct response in up to 86% of leukemia cells tested.

Historically, Brazilians have used acai berries to treat digestive disorders and skin conditions. Current marketing efforts suggest acai products can help consumers lose weight, lower cholesterol and gain energy. Because only recently the fruit has been available outside Brazil, very limited research has been done. So far, only fundamental research has been done on acai berries, which contain at least 50 to 75 unidentified compounds.

Acai is believed to have double the ORAC value of blueberries and 30 times that of red wine.

Bilberry

Bilberry, which is botanically related to blueberry, is a well known folk remedy for vision, and especially for night blindness. During WWII, Royal Air Force pilots were given bilberry jam as they claimed it significantly improved their visual acuity in the dark.

Bilberries contain anthocyanosides which are necessary for normal photosensitivies of the eyes and help them adapt to variations in light intensity. (Wegmann)

Anthocyanosides are antioxidants which have a strengthening effect of the walls of the small vessels and capillaries. (Scharrer, Lagrue, Bartolo, Mian)

Anthocyanosides have demonstrated ability to accelerate the production of rhodopsin (visual purple) in the retina. (Jayle) Visual purple is a pigment in the receptors in the eye needed to send nerve impulses to the brain. People who work with bright light (such as working in front of a computer) and suffer from eye fatigue can benefit from supplementation of anthocyanoside containing nutrients such as bilberry.

Blueberries (and other berries)

Blueberries, cranberries, strawberries, and raspberries all contain powerful disease fighting phytochemicals that fight (prevent and even reverse) cancer, heart disease, high cholesterol, stomach ulcers and more. Blueberries get very high ORAC scores... rating 2,400 per 100 grams. Researchers have counted almost 100 different phytochemicals, not to mention the dozens of vitamins, minerals and fiber blueberries provide. According to the USDA, these phytochemicals are analgesic, anti-bacterial, anti-cancer, anti-inflammatory, antioxidant, antiseptic, anti-sunburn, anti-ulcer and immunostimulants.

Imagine how many pharmaceuticals you would have to take to do all those things (but then have to suffer the side effects) - and it's all in just one yummy fruit.

Chlorella and Spirulina

Chlorella and Spirulina are so nutrient-rich, they are called "superfoods." These are both micro-algae that are now grown in fresh water farms but have existed since the Earth was in its earliest stages. Chlorella and Spirulina have been recognized for their seemingly limitless benefits they provide. These superfoods contain all essential amino acids, vitamins, minerals and fatty acids needed to sustain human life including other trace minerals, phytochemicals and other components that scientists haven't even identified yet. If you counted all the vitamins, minerals, fatty acids, enzymes, and phytochemicals in Chlorella or Spirulina, the number could be as high as 400!

Spirulina contains twelve times the digestible protein found in beef. Both Chlorella and Spirulina contain far more calcium than milk. Both have actually shrunk cancer tumors. They also regulate pH blood levels, which protects against loss of bone mass.

The nutritional substances in Chlorella and Spirulina are found in near perfect ratios and include: All eight essential amino acids, plus some non-essential, Vitamin A, all B's (including B-12 which is never found in plants), C, E, calcium, magnesium, zinc, potassium, dozens of trace minerals, Omega-3 fats, especially GLA, Mucopolysaccharides, Beta-Carotene, Nucleic Acids: RNA & DNA, Chlorophyll and hundreds of other phytochemicals.

The vitamin and mineral content of these superfoods are in their natural forms, the way the human body was meant to absorb them something which no man-made multi-vitamin or even regular vegetables can even compare.

CGF (chlorella growth factor), found in the nucleus of the chlorella cell, actually promotes the body's innate healing ability to grow and repair tissues. Studies show Chlorella's ability to fight tumors, viruses, and cancers are nothing short of remarkable. Chlorella increases the blood chemistry of the body by increasing red and white blood cells, platelets and albumin. People with cancer normally have a decreased level of albumin.

RNA/DNA are responsible for directing cellular renewal, growth, and repair. These nucleic acid levels in the body decrease with age and are depleted by lack of exercise, stress, pollution, and poor diet. Chlorella offers superior-quality RNA/DNA, measured by CGF, strengthens immunity by improving the activity of T- and B-cells, which defend against viruses and other invading microorganisms, and macrophages, which destroy cancer and cellular debris.

Spirulina contains potent anti-cancer phytochemicals that also gives spirulina its characteristic blue hue. These include: chlorophyll-a, xanthophyll, beta-carotene, echinenone, myxoxanthophyll, zeaxanthin, canthaxanthin, diatoxanthin, 3'-hydroxyechinenone, beta-cryptoxanthin, oscillaxanthin, plus the phycobilins c-phycocyanin and allophycocyanin.

The mucopolysaccharides found in spirulina and chlorella also support healthy intestinal flora, the "friendly" bacteria in your digestive tract.

Cruciferous Vegetables

The American Cancer Society, the National Cancer Institute and the National Institutes of Health all recommend that we eat more cruciferous vegetables to help prevent some forms of cancer, particularly gastrointestinal, respiratory tract and colo-rectal cancer. Studies also show that individuals who eat cruciferous vegetables also have lower rates of prostate and bladder cancers.

Cruciferous vegetables are the green leafy vegetables like **Broccoli, Cauliflower, Brussels Sprouts, Kale, Cabbage, Horseradish, Kohlrabi, and Mustard Greens.**

They contain a host of cancer-fighting, immune-promoting compounds, such as sulforaphane, indoles and isothiocyanates, which render carcinogens harmless.

Indoles enhance the body's detoxification abilities. One in particular, indole-3-carbonol, helps reduce the risk of breast cancer by acting as a precursor to estrogen. Indole-3-carbonol also inhibits chemically induced tumors in the forestomach, mammary gland, liver and inhibits estrogenic activity, reducing mammary tumors.

Sulforphane activates Phase II enzymes which tend to block formation of carcinogens or facilitate their excretion.

Cabbage and turnips also contain phenethy isothiocyanate which prevent enzymes from forming carcinogens from potentially harmful substances in our food, drink, and also smoke.

Cabbage and soy beans contain genistein. Genistein prevents the development of capillaries which form around a tumor. Without an adequate supply of oxygen and nutrients, the potential for tumor growth is impeded.

Cabbage also contains monoterpenes, which are cancer-fighting antioxidants that inhibit cholesterol production and provide other protective activities.

The sterols in cabbage protect us from breast cancer and block absorption of fats and cholesterol. Other foods containing sterols include broccoli, cucumbers, yams, sweet potatoes, squash, tomatoes, eggplant, peppers, and soy.

Green peppers, tomatoes, carrots and **strawberries** contain p-coumaric acid and chlorogenic acid which keep certain carcinogens from binding to the genetic material in cells, where they can cause damage.

Green Tea

Green Tea contains polyphenols which have antioxidant and anticarcinogenic properties.

The most important and most powerful polyphenol catechin is EGCG, which stands for epigallocatachin gallate. Green Tea Extract contains about 31% EGCG. This potent antioxidant is also an important element in the body's production of antibacterial factors, cholesterol stabilizers, and blood clotting substances. (Valcic)

Research has also demonstrated the beneficial protective relationship between green tea and cancer (Stoner, Cao), hypertension, tooth decay, gingivitis (Sakanaka), and cholesterol (Muramatsu). Much of the protective benefits in green tea stem from its ability to suppress free radical damage. (Stoner, Asano. Guo) Its antioxidant action is much stronger than both Vitamins C and E. (Zhao)

Grape Seed/Pine Bark Extract

Grape seed and pine bark extracts are very high in proanthocyanidins, which provide powerful antioxidant activities in the body.(Cheshier) Proanthocyanidins (a bioflavonoid) are believed to be the most potent form of antioxidants available in nature. Proanthocyanidins are actually 50 times more effective than Vitamin E and 20 times more effective than Vitamin C as an antioxidant. (Masquelier) At the same time proanthocyanidins give power to these so they work better together.

Proanthocyanidins protect us from free radical damage which contributes to cellular changes and invites degenerative diseases. Proanthocyanidins inhibit protease, enzymes which break down proteins. These enzymes are released in the body during inflammation. The inactivation of proteases may protect vascular walls in our vessels and capillaries. (Tixier, Rong, Bertuglia)

Proanthocyanidins strengthen the elasticity of connective tissue such as collagen and elastin (the connective tissues found in the joints and skin) Proanthocyanidins can help reduce cross linking. When there is excessive cross linking, the connective tissue becomes hard and inelastic. Cross linkages are the main cause of wrinkles and aging.

Proanthocyanidins regulate the release of histamine in the body. Histamine is responsible for many of the uncomfortable symptoms associated with allergies and colds. (Birkhauser, Verlog) Proanthocyanidins are also found in berries and other fruits and plants.

Mangosteen

Mangosteen (Garcinia Mangostana) is often called the "Queen of Fruits" because it taste great and has so many medicinal healing benefits. This fruit (about the size of a plum) contains the motherlode of the powerful antioxidant, xanthones. These antioxidants are found in a select number of rain forest plants, but nowhere are they found in more abundance than in the rind of the Mangosteen fruit. This smooth, purple covering ground up with ancient mortars was and is used to heal internal and external infections (great news for diabetics).

The two most beneficial xanthones found in the mangosteen are Alpha Mangostin and Gamma Mangostin. When isolated and thoroughly tested by researchers, these have been found to carry a host of benefits. According to professional journals such as *Free Radical Research, Journal of Pharmacology,* and the I*ndian Journal of Experimental Biology,* these xanthones have remarkable health benefits and are some of the most powerful antioxidants found in nature.

Red Wine

Red wine, like green tea, contains a powerful polyphenol, anthocyanes and in particular, one called malvoside. Researchers have shown a number of health promoting effects, including the cardiovascular system.

In countries where wine is the primary alcoholic drink, heart disease death rates are lowest. Interestingly, the opposite shows up for beer. Alcohol, in the amount of one glass per day, seems to elevate HDL "good" cholesterol.

Polyphenols in wine in addition to their antioxidant effects, also are antimicrobial. It is effective against cholera, the dreaded E. coli, and also E. typhi. The Greeks and others used to pour wine into wounds and over dressings to disinfect them.

The results of an international study suggests that a compound found in red wine gave mice longer and healthier lives and also countered some effects of a high-calorie diet.

My Healthiest Foods List

VEGETABLES

Alfalfa

Alfalfa contains saponins proven to help lower elevated cholesterol Researchers gave patients with elevated cholesterol 40 grams of alfalfa seeds three times daily. After eight weeks, their average total cholesterol was reduced by 17%, with an 18% reduction in LDL "bad" cholesterol.

Alfalfa sprouts are low in calories and fat, and high in fiber, trace minerals and enzymes - all eight essential enzymes. Alfalfa is also a good source of vitamin K, which facilitates blood clotting and helps to prevent hemorrhaging. Vitamin K also seems to help the body retain calcium and ward off osteoporosis.

Asparagus

A cup of asparagus supplies approximately 263 mcg of folate, a B-vitamin essential for proper cellular division because it is necessary in DNA synthesis and therefore very important to help prevent birth defects. Without folate, the fetus' nervous system cells do not divide properly. Inadequate folate during pregnancy has been linked to several birth defects, including neural tube defects like spina bifida.

Despite folate's wide availability in food (it's name comes from the Latin word folium, meaning "foliage," because it's found in green leafy vegetables), folate deficiency is <u>the most common vitamin deficiency</u> in the world.

Folate is also essential for a healthy cardiovascular system. Folate (along with vitamins B6 and B12) is necessary for the conversion of homocysteine into cysteine. When folate levels are low, blood levels of homocysteine rise--a situation that significantly increases the risk for heart disease. Homocysteine promotes atherosclerosis by reducing the integrity of blood vessel walls and by interfering with the formation of collagen (the main protein in connective tissue). Elevations in homocysteine are found in approximately 20-40% of patients with heart disease, and it is estimated that consumption of 400 mcg of folate daily would reduce the number of heart attacks suffered by Americans each year by 10%. Just one serving of asparagus supplies almost 60% of the daily recommended intake of folate!

Asparagus is a natural diuretic. It is a very good source of potassium (288 mg per cup) and low in sodium (19.8 mg per cup). Historically, asparagus has been used to treat inflammation, such as arthritis and rheumatism, and may also be useful for PMS-related water retention.

Asparagus contains a special insoluble fiber called inulin that health-promoting friendly bacteria in our large intestine love. Inulin supports the growth and activity of these friendly bacteria. And when populations of friendly bacteria are high, it is much more difficult for unfriendly bacteria to gain a foothold in our intestinal tract.

Avocados

These delicious fruits have gotten a bad reputation. Yes, they do contain fat and consequently a lot a calories, but they also contain Vitamins A, C and E, niacin, iron, and are very high in B-5, folic acid, potassium, and fiber. Almost all the fat in an avocado is unsaturated and of course, they contain no cholesterol.

Avocados contain oleic acid, a monounsaturated fat that may help to lower cholesterol. In one study of people with moderately high cholesterol levels, individuals who ate a diet high in avocados showed clear health improvements. After seven days on the diet that included avocados, they had significant decreases in total cholesterol and LDL cholesterol, along with an 11% increase in health promoting HDL cholesterol.

Avocados are a very good source of potassium, a mineral that helps regulate blood pressure. Adequate intake of potassium can help to guard against circulatory diseases, like high blood pressure, heart disease or stroke. One medium avocado has as much potassium as 3 bananas and more fiber than prunes! Avocados have the highest dietary fiber content on a weight basis of any fruit (1 gram per oz. and per 52 calories),

Beets

There's enough potassium in a serving of beets to help lower blood pressure and protect against stroke. They also contain manganese, calcium, and iron. A cup of cooked sliced beets has only 52 calories and a whopping 3.4 grams of fiber, about the same as 1 1/2 cups of cooked oatmeal.

Beets can also be eaten raw. Try them shredded on a salad and receive about twice the vitamin C as cooked ones.

Bell Peppers

Bell peppers (green, red, orange or yellow) are rich sources of vitamin C and beta-carotene, two very powerful antioxidants. These antioxidants work together to effectively neutralize free radicals.

For atherosclerosis and diabetic heart disease, peppers also contain vitamin B6 and folic acid.

Red peppers are one of the few foods that contain lycopene, a carotenoid whose consumption has been inversely correlated with prostate cancer and cancers of the cervix, bladder and pancreas. Recent studies suggest that individuals whose diets are low in lycopene-rich foods are at greater risk for developing these types of cancers.

Broccoli (Cauliflower, Brussels Sprouts, etc.)

These are cruciferous vegetables which contain phytochemicals--sulforaphane and the indoles--with significant anti-cancer effects. Research on indole-3-carbinol shows this compound helps deactivate a potent estrogen metabolite (4-hydroxyestrone) that promotes tumor growth, especially in estrogen-sensitive breast cells, while at the same time increasing the level of 2-hydroxyestrone, a form of estrogen that can be cancer-protective. Indole-3-carbinol not only suppresses breast tumor cell growth, but also metastasis (the movement of cancerous cells to other parts of the body).

Sulforaphane boosts the body's detoxification enzymes, potentially by altering gene expression, thus helping to clear potentially carcinogenic substances more quickly. When researchers at Johns Hopkins studied the effect of sulphoraphane on tumor formation in lab animals, those animals given sulforaphane had fewer tumors, and the tumors they did develop grew more slowly and weighed less, meaning they were smaller.

Additionally, researchers in the Netherlands investigated the effect of a diet high in brussels sprouts on DNA damage. They compared two groups of healthy male volunteers. Five men ate a diet that included about 10 ounces of cooked brussels sprouts daily, while the other five men at a diet free of cruciferous vegetables. After three weeks, the brussels sprouts group had 28% decrease in DNA damage. This may indicate a reduced risk of cancer since DNA mutations allow cancer cells to develop.

Sulforaphane can help stop the proliferation of breast cancer cells, even in the later stages of their growth. (*Journal of Nutrition*, September 2004)

Brussels sprouts' glucosinolates have been shown to help prevent the development of colon cancer in response to exposure to heterocyclic amines, the carcinogenic compounds produced when meat is grilled or otherwise charbroiled. In an animal study published in Carcinogenesis (Kassie F, Uhl M, et al., February 2003), researchers looked at the effects of drinking water supplemented with Brussels sprouts or red cabbage juices on the liver and colon of male rats that were also given a heterocyclic amine carcinogen.

Brussels sprouts reduced the development of pre-cancerous cells 41-52% in the colon and 27-67% in the liver, and drastically diminished the size (85-91%) of pre-cancerous lesions in the liver.

Cabbage

Much research has focused on the beneficial phytochemicals in cabbage, particularly its indole-3-carbinole (I3C), sulforaphane, and indoles. These two compounds help activate and stabilize the body's antioxidant and detoxification mechanisms that dismantle and eliminate cancer-producing substances. I3C has been shown to improve estrogen detoxification and to reduce the incidence of breast cancer.

Celery

Celery is an excellent source of vitamin C, a vitamin that helps to support the immune system. Vitamin C-rich foods like celery may help reduce cold symptoms or severity of cold symptoms; over 20 scientific studies have concluded that vitamin C is a cold-fighter. Vitamin C also prevents the free radical damage that triggers the inflammatory cascade, and is therefore also associated with reduced severity of inflammatory conditions, such as asthma, osteoarthritis, and rheumatoid arthritis. As free radicals can oxidize cholesterol and lead to plaques that may rupture causing heart attacks or stroke, vitamin C is beneficial to promoting cardiovascular health.

High blood pressure benefits: Celery contains active compounds called pthalides, which can help relax the muscles around arteries and allow those vessels to dilate. With more space inside the arteries, the blood can flow at a lower pressure. Pthalides also reduce stress hormones, one of whose effects is to cause blood vessels to constrict.

In animal studies, intake of the equivalent of 4 sticks of celery for humans was shown to lower the blood pressure by 12%. I tell people all the time: Eat four to five stalks of celery a day to fight high blood pressure... and they agree, it works!

Cucumbers

The flesh of cucumbers is primarily composed of water but also contains ascorbic acid (vitamin C) and caffeic acid, both of which help soothe skin irritations and reduce swelling. Cucumbers hard skin is rich in fiber and contains a variety of beneficial minerals including silica, potassium and magnesium.

The silica in cucumber is an essential component of healthy connective tissue, which includes intracellular cement, muscles, tendons, ligaments, cartilage, and bone. Cucumber juice is often recommended as a source of silicon to improve the complexion and health of the skin, plus cucumber's high water content makes it naturally hydrating--a must for glowing skin. Cucumbers are also used topically for various types of skin problems, including swelling under the eyes and sunburn. Two compounds in cucumbers, ascorbic acid and caffeic acid, prevent water retention, which may explain why cucumbers applied topically are often helpful for swollen eyes, burns and dermatitis.

Cucumber's high mineral content makes it extremely alkaline which helps to reduce an acidic system. This is important for high blood pressure, bone density and to support the immune system's fight against cancer, bacteria, viruses and candida.

Fennel

Fennel has its own unique combination of phytonutrients, including the flavonoids rutin, quercitin, and various kaempferol glycosides, all powerful antioxidants. The phytonutrients in fennel extracts combat BHT (butylated hydroxytoluene), a potentially toxic commonly added to processed foods.

The most fascinating phytonutrient compound in fennel, however, may be anethole. In animal studies, the anethole in fennel has repeatedly been shown to reduce inflammation and to help prevent the occurrence of cancer. Researchers have also proposed a biological mechanism that may explain these anti-inflammatory and anticancer effects. This mechanism involves the shutting down of a intercellular signaling system called tumor necrosis factor (or TNF)-mediated signaling. By shutting down this signaling process, the anethole in fennel prevents activation of a potentially strong gene-altering and inflammation-triggering molecule called NF-kappaB. The volatile oil has also been shown to be able to protect the liver of experimental animals from toxic chemical injury.

Garlic

A member of the lily or Allium family, which also includes onions, garlic is rich in a variety of powerful sulfur-containing compounds including thiosulfinates (of which the best known compound is allicin), sulfoxides (among which the best known compound is alliin), and dithiins (in which the most researched compound is ajoene). While these compounds are responsible for garlic's characteristically pungent odor, they are also the source of many of its health-promoting effects. In addition, garlic is an excellent source of manganese, a very good source of vitamin B6 and vitamin C and a good source of selenium.

Numerous studies have demonstrated that regular consumption of garlic lowers blood pressure, and decreases platelet aggregation, serum triglycerides and LDL-cholesterol (the potentially dangerous form) levels while increasing serum HDL-cholesterol (the protective form) and fibrinolysis (the process through which the body breaks up blood clots), and stimulating the production of nitric oxide in the lining of blood vessel walls, which helps them to relax. As a result of these beneficial actions, garlic helps prevent atherosclerosis and diabetic heart disease, and reduces the risk of heart attack or stroke.

Greens: Beet, turnip, mustard, collard, etc.

Greens are jam-packed with nutrients. They provide good to excellent amounts of 8+ vitamins, 10+ minerals, dietary fiber and protein. And if that were not enough, several of these are members of the Brassica family along with broccoli, cabbage and Brussels sprouts, so they also feature glucosinolates.

As excellent sources of three notable anti-oxidants:

vitamin E, vitamin C and vitamin A (through beta-carotene), these team up to scavenge free radicals. Beta-carotene and vitamin E exert their protective actions against free radicals in the lipid-soluble areas of the body, while vitamin C balances out the job by working in the body's water-soluble environment.

These are also excellent sources of vitamin K, needed for bone health and much more.

Kale

Kale's organosulfur compounds have been main subject of phytonutrient research, and these include the glucosinolates and the methyl cysteine sulfoxides. Although there are over 100 different glucosinolates in plants, only 10-15 are present in kale and other Brassicas. Yet these 10-15 glucosinolates appear able to lessen the occurrence of a wide variety of cancers, including breast and ovarian cancers. Researchers demonstrate the ability of its glucosinolates and cysteine sulfoxides to activate detoxifying enzymes in the liver that help neutralize potentially carcinogenic substances (quinone reductases and glutathione-S-transferases). These boost the body's detoxification processes, thus helping to clear potentially carcinogenic substances more quickly.

Sulforaphane triggers the liver to produce enzymes that detoxify cancer-causing chemicals, inhibits chemically-induced breast cancers in animal studies, induces colon cancer cells to commit suicide, and helps stop the proliferation of breast cancer cells, even in the later stages of their growth.

Sulforaphane may also offer special protection to those with colon cancer-susceptible genes, suggests a study conducted at Rutgers University and published online on May 4, 2006, in the journal *Carcinogenesis*.

Mushrooms

Mushrooms are very low in calories (1/2 cup of raw pieces has just 9 calories and 1/2 cup of cooked just 21).

Mushrooms are very high in potassium, low in sodium, and contain a fair amount of B vitamins.

Asian mushrooms are quickly gaining popularity for their ability to fight cancer, inhibit blood clotting, and stimulate immunity. Reishi mushrooms have anti-cancer and anti-histamine properties making them beneficial for individuals with allergies.

Shiitake mushrooms have been extensively researched. They contain lentinan, an anti-viral polysaccharide which stimulates the immune system to produce interferon which fights off cancerous cells. (Takehara) Lentinan is used as an anti-cancer treatment in Japan. Shiitake mushrooms may also help lower cholesterol.

Onions

Onions, like garlic, are members of the Allium family, and both are rich in powerful sulfur-containing compounds. Onions contain allyl propyl disulphide, while garlic is rich in allicin, diallyl disulphide, diallyl trisulfide and others. In addition, onions are very rich in chromium, a trace mineral that helps cells respond to insulin (excellent for diabetics!), plus vitamin C, and numerous flavonoids, most notably, quercitin (excellent for circulatory health and allergies).

Experimental and clinical evidence suggests that allyl propyl disulfide is responsible for this effect and lowers blood sugar levels by increasing the amount of free insulin available. Allyl propyl disulfide competes with insulin, which is also a disulphide, to occupy the sites in the liver where insulin is inactivated. This results is an increase in the amount of insulin available to usher glucose into cells causing a lowering of blood sugar.

Onions are also a very good source of chromium, the mineral component in glucose tolerance factor, a molecule that helps cells respond appropriately to insulin. Clinical studies of diabetics have shown that chromium can decrease fasting blood glucose levels, improve glucose tolerance, lower insulin levels, and decrease total cholesterol and triglyceride levels, while increasing good HDL-cholesterol levels. Marginal chromium deficiency is common in the United States, not surprising since chromium levels are depleted by consuming refined sugars, white flour products, and lack of exercise. One cup of raw onion contains almost 20% of the Daily Value of chromium.

The regular consumption of onions has, like garlic, been shown to lower high cholesterol levels and high blood pressure. This is likely due to onions' sulfur compounds, its chromium and its vitamin B6, which helps prevent heart disease by lowering high homocysteine levels, another significant risk factor for heart attack and stroke.

The regular use of onions (two+ per week) is associated with a significantly reduced risk of colon cancer. Onions contain a number of flavonoids, the most studied of which, quercitin, has been shown to halt the growth of tumors in animals and to protect colon cells from the damaging effects of certain cancer-causing substances. Cooking meats with onions may help reduce the carcinogens produced when meat is cooked in certain ways.

Parsley

Two types of unusual components provide unique health benefits: 1. Volatile oils, including myristicin, limonene, eugenol, and alpha-thujene. 2. Flavonoids, including apiin, apigenin, crisoeriol, and luteolin.

Parsley's volatile oils, particularly myristicin, have been shown to inhibit tumor formation in animal studies, and particularly, tumor formation in the lungs. Myristicin has also been shown to activate the enzyme glutathione-S-transferase, which helps attach the molecule glutathione to oxidized molecules that would otherwise do damage in the body. This activity qualifies it as a "chemoprotective" food, and in particular, a food that can help neutralize particular types of carcinogens (like the benzopyrenes that are part of cigarette smoke, charcoal grill smoke, and the smoke produced by trash incinerators).

Parsley's flavonoids, especially luteolin, combat free

radicals to help prevent damage to cells. In addition, extracts from parsley have been used in animal studies to help increase the anti-oxidant capacity of the blood.

In addition, parsley is an excellent source of three vital nutrients that are also important for the prevention of many diseases: vitamin C, beta-carotene, and folic acid.

Pumpkin

Yes! Pumpkin pie is actually good for us! Pumpkin, without the crust and whipped topping, is very low in calories, is loaded with beta carotene and fiber, and also contains vitamin C, calcium, magnesium, phosphorus, and more potassium than a banana (one cup pumpkin serving)!

Pumpkin seeds are noted for their high content of zinc, needed for wound healing, a healthy immune system, insulin production and male reproductive system. Pumpkin seed oil is recommended to men concerned about prostate health.

Pumpkin and **squash** (deep orange pulp like acorn) are very similar so they offer similar benefits, but squash also provides protease trypsin inhibitors that keep viruses and cancer-causing chemicals from becoming activated in the intestinal tract.

Sea Vegetables (Seaweed/Kelp)

There are many different types of edible seaweed, many of them referred to as kelp. In urban areas of Japan where seaweed consumption is dropping, cancer rates are rising compared to rural areas where seaweed consumption is high and cancer rates remain very low.

According to folklore, kelp was used to treat constipation, bronchitis, asthma, indigestion, ulcers, colitis, gallstones, obesity, arthritis, and to combat stress, skin diseases and insect bites. Hard to believe, but scientists have confirmed that seaweed contains valuable health promoting phytonutrients such as fucoidan polysaccharides which demonstrate antitumor activity in mice. (Zhuang) Research suggests that the antitumor activity of fucoidan is related to the enhancement of immune responses. (Itoh)

Brown algal-sulfated polysaccharides have anti-clotting activities and ability to reduce LDL cholesterol and increase HDL cholesterol. Scientists have also isolated blood-pressure lowering compounds in seaweed such as histamine. Therefore seaweed is an excellent choice to help maintain heart health.

Kelp is also a good source of iodine, essential for the thyroid. Iodine deficiency can result in weight gain, extreme fatigue, and feeling cold all the time.

Spinach

Spinach researchers have identified at least 13 different flavonoid compounds in spinach that function as antioxidants and as anti-cancer agents (methylenedioxyflavonol glucuronides.) The anticancer properties of these spinach flavonoids have been sufficiently impressive to prompt researchers to create specialized spinach extracts that could be used in controlled studies. These spinach extracts have been shown to slow down cell division in stomach cancer cells (gastric adenocarcinomas), and in studies on mice, to reduce skin cancers. A study on adult women living in New England in the late 1980s also showed intake of spinach to be inversely related to incidence of breast cancer.

Spinach Carotenoid Combats Prostate Cancer: A carotenoid found in spinach and other green leafy vegetables fights human prostate cancer two different ways, according to research published in the September 2004 issue of the *Journal of Nutrition*. The carotenoid, called neoxanthin, not only induces prostate cancer cells to self-destruct, but is converted in the intestines into additional compounds, called neochromes, which put prostate cancer cells into a state of stasis, thus preventing their replication. (December 13, 2004)

Popeye may have made himself strong by eating spinach, but he may also have been protecting himself against osteoporosis, heart disease, colon cancer, arthritis, and other diseases at the same time.

The vitamin K provided by spinach, almost 200% of the Daily Value in one cup of fresh spinach leaves and over 1000% of the Daily Value in one cup of boiled spinach (containing about 6 times more spinach) is important for maintaining bone health. Vitamin K1 activates osteocalcin, the major non-collagen protein in bone. Osteocalcin anchors calcium molecules inside of the bone. Therefore, without enough vitamin K1, osteocalcin levels are inadequate, and bone mineralization is impaired.

Tomatoes

Lycopene is the primary carotenoid found in tomatoes (and everything made from them). It has been extensively studied for its antioxidant and cancer-preventing properties. Lycopene helps protect cells and other structures in the body from oxygen damage, including protection of DNA (our genetic material) inside of white blood cells. Prevention of heart disease has been shown to be another antioxidant role played by lycopene.

Lycopene from tomatoes has been repeatedly studied in humans and found to be protective against a growing list of cancers, now including colorectal, prostate, breast, endometrial, lung, and pancreatic cancers.

For the most lycopene, choose organic: Organic ketchup delivers three times as much of the cancer-fighting carotenoid, lycopene, as non-organic brands.

Lycopene has been shown to help protect not only against prostate, but breast, pancreatic and intestinal cancers, especially when consumed with fat-rich foods, such as avocado, olive oil or nuts. (Carotenoids are fat-soluble, meaning they are absorbed into the body along with fats.) For this reason, cooked tomatoes (as is marinara sauce, pizza sauce, etc. which is usually cooked with olive oil provides an excellent source for lycopene.

Yams/Sweet Potatoes

These are so good for us its a shame that so many only enjoy them a few times a year during the holidays.

These two similar tubers (edible root-like structures) are rich in plant sterols which are fat-like compounds block estrogen promotion of breast cancer activity, and help block the absorption of cholesterol.

Dioscorea yams are known to contain a high amount of a progesterone-like substance believed to help many women's problems such as PMS and menopause.

It is suspected that hormone-like substances in the yam stimulate the ovaries to release more than one egg. These hormone-like substances deserve more research to determine their full potential.

Sweet potatoes contain a number of polyphenol compounds, such as chlorogenic acid, which work together to create a powerful antioxidant effect.

Sweet potatoes are rich in natural protease inhibitors that prevent the spread of cancer in animal studies and have become popular for their ability to kill disease producing viruses such as HIV.

Sweet potatoes are full of fiber which also helps us fight off cancer, maintain good colon health, and help us keep excess weight off. They are also very high in the antioxidant beta carotene, and very high in potassium, magnesium, and folic acid.

FRUITS

Acia Berries - *see page 18.*

Apples

Apples feature fiber, flavonoids and fructose that makes the saying, "An apple a day, keep the doctor away" really true!

Apples contain both insoluble and soluble fiber. One medium unpeeled apple provides over 3 grams of fiber. Apple's two types of fiber pack a double punch that can knock down cholesterol levels, reducing your risk of hardening of the arteries, heart attack, and stroke. Apple's insoluble fiber works like bran, latching on to LDL cholesterol in the digestive tract and removing it from the body, while apple's soluble fiber pectin reduces the amount of LDL cholesterol produced in the liver. Eating just one large apple has been shown to decrease serum cholesterol 8-11%. Eating 2 large apples a day has lowered cholesterol levels by up to 16%!

A flavonoid pigment in apples that helps provide their color have been extensively researched and found to help prevent heart disease.

Apple skin and onions are the two major food sources of a potent antioxidant flavonoid called quercitin. Quercitin is especially beneficial when teamed up with another antioxidant, vitamin C, also found in apples, to boost our immune defenses. This dynamic antioxidant duo provides another way (in addition to fiber) through which apples protect against cancer and also helps prevent the free radical damage to LDL cholesterol that promotes heart disease.

Apple peel contains high concentrations of special antioxidant compounds called phenols that may assist in the prevention of a number of chronic diseases. Now it appears that the phenols in the skin of certain cultivars of apples may provide a hefty dose of UV-B protection, according to a study published in the August 2003 issue of the *Journal of Experimental Botany*.

Apricots

Nutrients in apricots can help protect the heart and eyes, as well as provide the disease-fighting effects of fiber. The high beta-carotene and lycopene activity of apricots makes them important heart health foods. Both beta-carotene and lycopene protect LDL cholesterol from oxidation, which may help prevent heart disease.

Apricots contain nutrients such as Vitamin A that promote good vision. Vitamin A, a powerful antioxidant, quenches free radical damage to cells and tissues. Free radical damage can injure the eyes' lenses.

Bananas

Bananas are one of our best sources of potassium, an essential mineral for maintaining normal blood pressure and heart function. The average banana contains 467 mg of potassium and only 1 mg of sodium, so a banana a day may help to prevent high blood pressure and protect against atherosclerosis. Also, if you ever experience heart burn, try eating part of a banana for fast relief!

Bananas are an exceptionally rich source of fructooligosaccharide, a prebiotic compound which nourishes probiotic (friendly) bacteria in the colon. These beneficial bacteria produce vitamins and digestive enzymes that improve our ability to absorb nutrients, plus compounds that protect us against unfriendly microorganisms. When fructooligosaccharides are fermented by these friendly bacteria, not only do numbers of probiotic bacteria increase, but so does the body's ability to absorb calcium. In addition, gastrointestinal transit time is lessened, decreasing the risk of colon cancer.

Blackberries

An extract derived from fresh blackberries has shown to reduce cancerous tumors and prevent the proliferation of cancer cells in animal models. The water-soluble flavonoid cyanidin-3-glucoside (C3G) is the active compound responsible for blackberries' antioxidant benefits.

Blackberries also protect against the negative effects of carcinogenic HAs (heterocyclic amines). So far, there are 20 of them identified, which are created in some heated foods, such as fried meats. Several recent epidemiological studies show a correlation between the intake of fried meat and the development of cancer in the large intestine, breast and prostate.

Preliminary findings suggest that plant foods protect us. Among the most effective of these protectors were extracts from green tea, red wine, blueberries, blackberries, red grapes, kiwi, watermelon, parsley and spinach.

Blueberries *(also see page 18)*

Blueberries are literally bursting with nutrients and flavor, yet very low in calories. Recently, researchers at Tufts University analyzed 60 fruits and vegetables for their antioxidant capability. Blueberries came out on top, rating highest in their capacity to destroy free radicals.

Blueberries are packed with antioxidant phytonutrients called anthocyanidins, blueberries neutralize free radical damage to the collagen matrix of cells and tissues that can lead to cataracts, glaucoma, varicose veins, hemorrhoids, peptic ulcers, heart disease and cancer. Anthocyanins, the blue-red pigments found in blueberries, improve the integrity of support structures in the veins and entire vascular system. Anthocyanins enhance the effects of vitamin C, improve capillary integrity, and stabilize the collagen matrix (the ground substance of all body tissues). They prevent free-radical damage, inhibit enzymes from cleaving the collagen matrix, and directly cross-link with collagen fibers to form a more stable collagen matrix.

Cocoa Beans

Yes, I know, you are all SHOCKED to see cocoa beans in the fruit section! Technically, cocoa beans are are the seeds of the Theobroma tree (originally found in South and Central America). Cocoa pods (6-12 inches long) are the fruit of the cocoa tree. Each fruit carries between 30 and 40 beans. Chocolate and cocoa powder are derived from these beans. Cocoa contains the highest capacity of the antioxidant procyanidin.

Cocoa's antioxidant flavanols (flavan-3-ols) have been linked to lower blood pressure and improved function of the cells lining the blood vessels, offering extraordinary cardiovascular protection. Participants in a study of flavanol-rich cocoa showed improved blood vessel function after consuming a cocoa beverage, researchers from Harvard Medical School and the Brigham and Women's Hospital in Boston found. (*Arch Intern Med.* 2006)

Natural cocoa powders contain the highest levels of TAC and procyanidins. Milk chocolates, which contain the least amount of cocoa solids, have the lowest TAC and procyanidin levels. Baking chocolates contain fewer procyanidins, because they contain more fat (50-60%) than natural cocoa. Alkalinization, used to reduce the acidity and raise the pH of cocoa (Dutch chocolate), markedly reduces procyanidin content. Higher amounts of cocoa ingredients have higher procyanidin contents, and therefore, have higher antioxidant capacities.

Note: In baking I use 100% cocoa powder and sweeten it with stevia (an herb available in powder or liquid extract form) which has no calories, no effect on blood sugar and no negative effects on the immune system. I sometimes use honey (also made by God)...but it does have calories and does raise blood sugar. (*It is not good to eat much honey: so for men to search their own glory is not glory.* Proverbs 25:27)

Cranberries

Cranberries are low-calorie (low sugar) fruit that is rich in vitamin C and high in antioxidants.

As a rule, fruits contain approximately twice as many antioxidant phenols as vegetables. But, for cranberries, the the phenol content is was five times that of broccoli. The cranberry is one of North America's three native fruits that are commercially harvested. Its history can be traced back to this country's infancy, when it was used by the native Americans to relieve aches and pains. Today, studie show that cranberries can help prevent urinary tract infections and may reduce the risk of gum disease, stomach ulcers and cancer.

Hippuric acid in cranberries are natural antibiotics in the body. It survives the digestive tract and ends up in the urine where it can fight off bacterial agents. (Soboto) Studies show improvement in 70% of the women and men drinking 16 oz. of cranberry juice for 21 days for acute urinary tract infections. The stronger the juice, the more powerful the effect. Cranberry juice cocktail available at the grocery store is only about 25 to 35% pure berry juice (and look out for added sugars!). 100% juice concentrate is available at most health food stores.

The acidic effect that cranberry juice has on the urine is also helpful to prevent kidney stones.

Other foods which provide a natural antibiotic effect include **apples, buckwheat, chili peppers, water chestnuts, eggs, garlic, ginger, honey, hops, milk (raw), onions, radishes and tea.**

Figs

Figs contain Benzaldehyde, which provides antitumor activity. In one study with 65 patients with inoperable cancer in the advanced stages given Benzaldehyde 55% responded favorably; seven patients achieved complete recovery, 29 achieved partial improvement, 24 remained stable, and only five showed progression of the disease. (Kochi) In the Old Testament, Isaiah called for figs to heal King Hezekiah who was "sick unto death" from "a boil," which was probably cancer. The king recovered. Figs also contain antibacterial, antiparasitic enzymes called ficins that aid digestion.

Grapefruit

Grapefruit is an excellent source of vitamin C, a vitamin that helps to support the immune system. Vitamin C-rich foods like grapefruit may help reduce cold symptoms or severity of cold symptoms; over 20 scientific studies have suggested that vitamin C is a cold-fighter. Vitamin C also prevents the free radical damage that triggers the inflammatory cascade, and is therefore also associated with reduced severity of inflammatory conditions, such as asthma, osteoarthritis, and rheumatoid arthritis. As free radicals can oxidize cholesterol and lead to plaques that may rupture causing heart attacks or stroke, vitamin C also promotes cardiovascular health. Research shows that consumption of vegetables and fruits high in this nutrient (C) is associated with a reduced risk of death from all causes including heart disease, stroke and cancer.

The rich pink and red colors of grapefruit are due to

lycopene, a carotenoid phytochemical, which appears to have anti-tumor activity. Among the common dietary carotenoids, lycopene has the highest capacity to help fight free radicals, which can damage cells.

Grapefruit limonoids inhibit tumor formation by promoting the formation of glutathione-S-transferase, a detoxifying enzyme. This enzyme sparks a reaction in the liver that helps to make toxic compounds more water soluble for excretion from the body. Pulp of citrus like grapefruit contain glucarates, which may help prevent breast cancer.

Limonoids may also help fight cancers of the mouth, skin, lung, breast, stomach and colon. Our bodies readily absorb and utilize a very long-acting limonoid called limonin that is present is citrus fruits in about the same amount as vitamin C.

Grapes and Raisins

Grapes contain loads of beneficial flavonoids, which give the vibrant purple color to grapes, grape juice and red wine; the stronger the color, the higher the concentration of flavonoids. These flavonoid compounds include quercitin, as well resveratrol. Both appear to decrease the risk of heart disease by:

• Reducing platelet clumping and harmful blood clots

• Protecting LDL cholesterol from the free radical damage that initiates LDL's artery-damaging actions

Grapes and products made from grapes, such as wine and grape juice, may protect the French from their high-fat diets. Diets high in saturated fats like butter and lard, and lifestyle habits like smoking are risk factors for heart disease. Yet, French people with these habits have a lower risk of heart attack than Americans do. One clue that may help explain this "French paradox" is their frequent consumption of grapes and red wines.

Researchers found several beneficial effects from grape juice consumption. First, an increase occurred in levels of nitric oxide, a compound produced in the body that helps reduce the formation of clots in blood vessels.

Second, a decrease occurred in platelet aggregation, or blood clotting, by red blood cells. Lastly, researchers saw an increase in levels of alpha-tocopherol (vitamin E), which increased blood plasma antioxidant activity by 50%.

Grape juice also protected LDL cholesterol from oxidation, which turns LDL into an artery-damaging molecule. (LDL is often called the "bad" form of cholesterol, but it is actually benign and only becomes harmful after it is damaged by free radicals or "oxidized."

Phenolic compounds in grape skins inhibit enzymes that play a key role in cell regulation and also suppress the production of endothelin-1 (ET-1) that causes blood vessels to constrict, thus reducing the flow of oxygen to the heart. ET-1 is thought to contribute to the development of heart disease. Resveratrol prevents the expression of ET-1, at least in part, by significantly lessening free radical formation (which can result from stress).

Resveratrol helps keep the heart muscle flexible and healthy. It inhibits angiotensin II, a hormone that is secreted in response to high blood pressure and heart failure.

Kiwi

Kiwi has an interesting ability to protect DNA in the nucleus of human cells from oxygen-related damage. Researchers are not even certain which compounds in kiwi give it this protective antioxidant capacity, but they are sure that this healing property is not limited to those nutrients most commonly associated with kiwi, including its vitamin C or beta-carotene content. Since kiwi contains a variety of flavonoids and carotenoids that have demonstrated antioxidant activity, these phytonutrients in kiwi may be responsible for this DNA protection.

Kiwi also protects against respiratory health problems: wheezing, shortness of breath, or night coughing.

Kiwi is an excellent source of vitamin C and a good source of two of the most important fat-soluble antioxidants, vitamins E and A (in the form of beta-carotene). Kiwi is also a very good source of dietary fiber which can reduce high cholesterol levels, and may reduce the risk of heart disease and heart attack. Fiber is also good for binding and removing toxins from the colon, which is helpful for preventing colon cancer. In addition, fiber-rich foods, like kiwi, are good for keeping blood sugar levels under control. Kiwi also is a good source of potassium, magnesium, copper and phosphorous.

Lemon/Limes

Lemons and limes are an excellent source of Vitamin C and contain unique flavonoid compounds with antioxidant and anti-cancer properties. In limes, flavonoids called flavonol glycosides have been shown to stop cell division in many cancer cell lines. But, they are perhaps most interesting for their antibiotic effects. In several villages in West Africa where cholera epidemics had occurred, the inclusion of lime juice during the main meal of the day was determined to have been protective against the contraction of cholera. (Cholera is a disease triggered by activity of the Vibrio cholera bacteria). Lime juice was strongly protective effect against cholera.

Lemon and lime juice alter cell cycles (including the decision a cell makes about whether to divide or die) and the activities of immune cells called monocytes.

In animal studies and laboratory tests with human cells, compounds in citrus fruits, including lemons and limes, called limonoids have been shown to help fight cancers of the mouth, skin, lung, breast, stomach and colon. Now, scientists from the US Agricultural Research Service have shown that our bodies can readily absorb and utilize a very long-acting limonoid called limonin that is present is citrus fruits in about the same amount as vitamin C.

Traces of limonin can often still be detected 24 hours after consumption! Other natural anti-carcinogens are available for much less time; for example, the phenols in green tea and chocolate remain active in the body for just 4 to 6 hours. Researchers are also investigating the potential cholesterol-lowering effects of limonin.

Pears

Pears contain ellagic acid which neutralizes carcinogens in the gastrointestinal tract before they can cause damage. (Barch, Harttig)

Pineapple

Pineapple contains bromelain, a proteolytic enzyme. Proteolytic enzymes, also called protease, aid in the breakdown of protein. Bromelain is a commonly used digestive aid. As we get older we produce fewer digestive enzymes making it more difficult to breakdown our food and also making us feel uncomfortable after eating, especially a meal high in protein. Raw pineapple may be an excellent desert choice which will actually help you digest your meal!

Protease enzymes also stimulate the immune system cells. They can aid in the destruction of collagen cross linkages (from free radicals) that form wrinkles and hardening of the arteries. According to the free radical theory of aging, it is cross linkages that essentially break down the cellular structure throughout the body causing degeneration.

Is Pineapple a Hawaiian Anti-aging Secret? It is interesting that in areas where pineapple is consumed abundantly, such as Hawaii, the people do not show the signs of aging that one might expect would accompany their high exposure to the sun. Might this be due to bromelains potential to ward off wrinkles?

Bromelain and other protease enzymes, interferes with arachidonic acid metabolism, which is involved in inflammation. Bromelain, with vitamin C and bioflavonoids, can be more effective than aspirin and other nonsteroidal anti-inflammatory drugs, for reducing pain and swelling of arthritis, sports injuries. (Lotz-Winter) Bromelain is also helpful for allergies and other inflammatory conditions.

Bromelain also has antiplatelet clotting activities. (Vellini) Heat destroys enzymes so pineapple must be eaten raw to obtain these excellent benefits of the bromelain.

Pineapple also contains potassium, lots of vitamin C, fiber, and manganese.

Another excellent source of protease enzymes is **papaya** which contains papain. Papaya is also rich in vitamin C, beta carotene, and potassium. In fact, papaya juice has 3 times more vitamin C and 22 times more vitamin A than orange juice! Something to remember the next time you think you are coming down with a cold or flu.

Plums and Prunes

The fresh version (plums) and the dried version (prunes) provide a high content of unique phytonutrients called neochlorogenic and chlorogenic acid. These substances found in plum and prune are classified as phenols, and their function as antioxidants is well-documented.

Phenols are very effective in neutralizing superoxide anion radicals, a particularly destructive free radical, and they have also been shown to help prevent oxygen-based damage to fats, such as the fats that make up a substantial portion of our brain cells or neurons, the cholesterol and triglycerides circulating in our bloodstream, or that make up our cell membranes.

Pomegranates

Antioxidants in pomegranates include polyphenols, such as tannins and anthocyanins. Pomegranates may have more antioxidant power than cranberry juice or green tea.

Pomegranate juice may improve blood flow to the heart in people with ischemic coronary heart disease (CHD). In a study of 45 people with CHD and myocardial ischemia (in which not enough blood gets to the heart muscle), participants who drank about 8 fluid ounces of pomegranate juice daily for 3 months had less ischemia during a stress test. Study participants who did not drink the juice, meanwhile, had evidence of more stress-induced ischemia. The study noted no negative effects to drinking pomegranate juice (even on blood sugar levels or body weight).

Pomegranate juice may help stop plaque from building up in blood vessels, having an anti-atherogenic effect. The antioxidants in the juice may help keep cholesterol in a form that is less damaging, and may also reduce plaque that has already built up in vessels. Pomegranate juice has shown to decrease the likelihood of LDL "bad" cholesterol to form plaque.

Pomegranate juice may slow prostate cancer growth. Antioxidants are known to help prevent and repair DNA damage that can lead to cancer. Men who have already had preliminary treatment for prostate cancer may benefit from a daily dose of pomegranate juice. The juice appeared to suppress the growth of cancer cells and the increase in cancer cell death in lab testing, according to research from UCLA. The combination of elements in pomegranates, rather than any single component, is probably responsible for it's excellent health effects.

Strawberries and Raspberries

Strawberries and raspberries contain ellagic acid which neutralizes carcinogens in the gastrointestinal tract before they can cause damage. (Barch, Harttig)

BEANS & LEGUMES

Beans and lentils contain phytates which appear to ward off cancer. Lentils and other legumes are a terrific source of soluble and insoluble fiber: 1/2 cup serving bas 3.7 grams of dietary fiber. Lentils are also high in protein, and low in fat and calories. Lentils are exceptionally high in folic acid and also contain potassium, iron, and copper.

Soluble fiber bas been shown to reduce blood cholesterol levels, which reduces the risk of diabetes and cardiovascular disease. Soluble fiber promotes bowel regularity by decreasing transit time. This form of fiber is believed to reduce the risk of developing colon cancer.

Black Beans

While beans are noted as a rich source of fiber nd low-fat source of protein, research indicates that black beans are just as rich in anthocyanins as grapes and cranberries, fruits long considered antioxidant superstars.

When researchers analyzed different types of beans, they found that, the darker the bean's seed coat, the higher its level of antioxidant activity. Gram for gram, black beans have the most antioxidant activity, followed in descending order by red, brown, yellow, and white beans.

Overall, the level of antioxidants found in black beans is approximately 10 times that found in an equivalent amount of oranges, and comparable to that found in an equivalent amount of grapes or cranberries.

Soybeans and Tofu contain isoflavon, phytoestrogens that mimic the action of estrogen in humans. While phyto-estrogens can act like estrogen, they are without any of the negative aspects. Women in Japan, where soy products are eaten almost daily, do not suffer from breast cancer and menopausal symptoms such as hot flashes, which are quite common among Western women.

Japanese men, because of their high soy diet, also have lower rates of prostate cancer than Western men.

Another beneficial compound in soy, genistein, blocks the growth of new capillaries that supply blood to some tumors, thus starving them of nutrients. Genistein may help to prevent the spread of cancer.

Soybeans are an excellent source of lecithin, a complex mixture of phospholipids consisting of essential fatty acids, choline, inositol and phosphorus. It is present in both animal and vegetable cells and is capable of emulsifying fats and water. One of the most important functions of lecithin concerns the control of cholesterol and other fats in the body. Lecithin helps us burn fats. Without it we can end up with gall stones and worse. Soy lecithin is an important source of essential polyunsaturated fatty acids.

Other foods containing lecithin include wheat germ oil, some nuts and seeds and egg yolks. If you do not break the yolk while cooking (such as soft boiled or poached) you protect the lecithin and avoid creating trans fatty acids.

NUTS & SEEDS

Almonds

Almonds are high in monounsaturated fats, the same type of health-promoting fats as are found in olive oil, which have been associated with reduced risk of heart disease.

Almonds' ability to reduce heart disease risk may also be partly due to its antioxidant action of vitamin E, as well as to the LDL-lowering effect of almonds' monounsaturated fats. (LDL is the "bad" form of cholesterol). When almonds are substituted for more traditional fats in human feeding trials, LDL cholesterol can be reduced from 8 to 12%.

A quarter-cup of almonds contains almost 98 mg of magnesium (24.7% of the daily value), plus 257 mg of potassium. Magnesium and potassium are important for electrolyte balance, blood pressure, nerve transmission and the contraction of all muscles including the heart. Almonds, therefore. help protect against high blood pressure and atherosclerosis (raw and unsalted).

The flavonoids found in almond skins team up with the vitamin E found in their meat to more than double the antioxidant punch either delivers when administered separately. (*Journal of Nutrition*, June 2005)

Twenty potent antioxidant flavonoids has been identified in almond skins. Blood tests demonstrated that eating almonds with their skins significantly increases both flavonoids and vitamin E in the body. While almond skin flavonoids alone enhanced LDL's resistance to oxidation by 18%, when almond meat's vitamin E was added, LDL's resistance to oxidation was extended by 52.5%! The synergy between the flavonoids and vitamin E in almonds demonstrates how the nutrients in whole foods such as almonds can impact health.

Almonds are good sources of manganese and copper, two trace minerals essential cofactors of a key oxidative enzyme, superoxide dismutase. This disarms free radicals produced within the mitochondria (the energy production factories within our cells), thus keeping our energy flowing.

Flax Seed

Flax is a small grain which contains the highest known vegetarian source of Omega-3 (alpha-linolenic acid). One serving (20 grams) of flax contains: 3,200 mg. Omega-3 fatty acids, plus 6 grams of fiber of which 1,600 micrograms are cancer-fighting lignans.

Of the 45 essential nutrients that must be obtained from foods, two are fatty acids: Omega-6 (linoleic acid), a polyunsaturated EFA; and Omega-3 (alpha-linolenic acid), a superunsaturated EFA.

Omega-3 is vital to brain development, normal blood pressure, healthy skin and an effective immune system. Omega-3 fatty acids lower triglycerides and at high levels, lower cholesterol. The anti-aggregatory, anti-thrombotic and anti-inflammatory properties of Omega-3 in the body have been clinically demonstrated.

Omega-3 oils break down into EPA (eicosapentaenoic acid) and DHA (docohexaenoic acid). EPA specifically plays an important role in heart health. DHA has been linked to brain health (memory, depression, etc.).

These two EFAs form the membranes of every one of the billions of cells in our bodies. They are also needed for cellular energy production and hormone production, such as prostaglandins. They are the raw materials to prostaglandins, which regulate or control the following:

* Inflammatory process
* Healing and repair
* Immune system
* Neural circuits in the brain
* Cardiovascular system including cholesterol
* Blood pressure
* Blood coagulation
* Digestive and reproductive systems
* Body thermostat and calorie-burning
* Cell growth and proliferation

Flaxseed is nature's richest source of lignans (also found in bran, buckwheat, corn, etc). Lignans deactivate potent estrogens that can initiate the growth of cancerous tumors, especially in the breast and reproductive system. In fact, studies show women who consume a diet high in lignans have lower rates of colon and breast cancer.

Pumpkin Seeds

Pumpkin seeds may promote prostate health. One factor that contributes to BPH is the overstimulation of prostate cells by testosterone and its conversion product, DHT (dihydrotestosterone). Components in pumpkin seed oil appear able to interrupt this triggering of prostate cell multiplication by testosterone and DHT.

The prostate-helpful components found in the oil extracts are found in the whole seeds; but it is unknown whether the amount of seeds eaten for a normal snack would contain enough to support the prostate.

The carotenoids and the omega-3 fats found in pumpkin seeds are also being studied for their potential prostate benefits. Men with higher amounts of carotenoids in their diet have less risk for BPH; this is the connection that has led to an interest in pumpkin seed carotenoids. The zinc found in pumpkin seeds may also benefit prostate function.

Zinc-rich foods, such as pumpkin seeds, also supports bone mineral density.

Pumpkin seeds also contain phytosterols which lower cholesterol. Phytosterols are compounds found in plants that have a chemical structure very similar to cholesterol, and when present in the diet in sufficient amounts, are believed to reduce blood levels of cholesterol, enhance the immune response and decrease risk of certain cancers.

Walnuts

This delicious nut is an excellent source of omega-3 essential fatty acids, a special type of protective fat the body cannot manufacture. Walnuts' concentration of omega-3s (a quarter-cup provides 90.8% of the daily value for these essential fats) has many potential health benefits: cardiovascular protection, better brain function, anti-inflammatory benefits for asthma, rheumatoid arthritis, and inflammatory skin diseases such as eczema and psoriasis. In addition, walnuts contain an antioxidant compound called ellagic acid that supports the immune system and appears to have several anticancer properties.

Walnuts are also an important source of monounsaturated fats-- approximately 15% of the fat found in walnuts is healthful monounsaturated fat. Studies have shown that increasing the dietary intake of monounsaturated-dense walnuts has favorable effects on high cholesterol levels and other cardiovascular risk factors.

GRAINS

Amaranth

Amaranth, known as the grain of the Aztecs. It is a small seed that resembles millet. It has a mild, nutty flavor. Amaranth can be eaten as a cereal, used in bread, added to soups or salad or eaten as a main dish.

Amaranth is rich in lysine, one of the eight essential amino acids, which is usually missing in plant food (but is abundant in animal protein). Amaranth is high in iron and calcium. A 2-ounce serving of cooked amaranth contains 80% of the RDA for iron and 10% of the RDA for calcium. Amaranth is also low in fat and calories and high in fiber.

Barley

Barley is a very good source of fiber and selenium, and a good source of phosphorus, copper and manganese.

Barley's dietary fiber also provides food for the "friendly" bacteria in the large intestine. When these helpful bacteria ferment barley's insoluble fiber, they produce a short-chain fatty acid called butyric acid, which serves as the primary fuel for the cells of the large intestine and helps maintain a healthy colon. These helpful bacteria also create two other short-chain fatty acids, propionic and acetic acid, which are used as fuel by the cells of the liver and muscles.

The propionic acid from barley's insoluble fiber may also be partly responsible for the cholesterol-lowering properties. In addition, barley is high in beta glucan, which helps to lower cholesterol by binding to bile acids and removing them from the body via the feces. Bile acids are used to digest fat that are manufactured by the liver from cholesterol. When they are excreted along with barley's fiber, the liver must manufacture new bile acids and uses up more cholesterol, thus lowering the amount of cholesterol in circulation. Soluble fiber may also reduce the amount of cholesterol manufactured by the liver.

Studies suggests barley's fiber has multiple beneficial effects on cholesterol with a significant ability to lower total cholesterol, plus increase large LDL and large and intermediate HDL fractions (which are considered less atherogenic) increased, and decrease the smaller LDL and VLDL cholesterol (the most dangerous fractions).

Buckwheat

Buckwheat provides a rich supply of flavonoids, particularly rutin, which protect against disease by extending the action of vitamin C and acting as antioxidants. Buckwheat's lipid-lowering activity is largely due to rutin and other flavonoid compounds. These compounds help maintain blood flow, keep platelets from clotting excessively (platelets are compounds in blood that, when triggered, clump together, thus preventing excessive blood loss, and protect LDL from free radical oxidation into potentially harmful cholesterol oxides. All these actions help to protect against heart disease.

Buckwheat also contains almost 86 milligrams of magnesium in a one cup serving. Magnesium relaxes blood vessels, improving blood flow and nutrient delivery while lowering blood pressure--the perfect combination for a healthy cardiovascular system.

The nutrients in buckwheat may contribute to blood

sugar control. When researchers followed almost 36,000 women in Iowa during a six-year long study of the effects of whole grains and the incidence of diabetes, they found that women who consumed an average of 3 servings of whole grains daily had a 21% lower risk of diabetes compared to those who ate one serving per week. Because buckwheat is an excellent source of magnesium, it is also important to note that women who ate the most foods high in magnesium had a 24% lower risk of diabetes compared to women who ate the least.

Oats

Oats, oat bran, and oatmeal contain a specific type of fiber known as beta-glucan. Since 1963, study after study has proven the beneficial effects of this special fiber on cholesterol levels. Studies show that in individuals with high cholesterol (above 220 mg/dl), consuming just 3 grams of soluble oat fiber per day (an amount found in one bowl of oatmeal) can lower total cholesterol up to 23%.

Beta-glucan is also beneficial for diabetics. Type 2 diabetes patients given foods high in oat fiber or given oatmeal or oat-bran rich foods experienced much lower rises in blood sugar compared to those who were given white rice or bread. Blood-sugar-stabilizing foods such as oats eaten in morning may make it easier to keep blood sugar levels under control the rest of the day.

Antioxidant compounds unique to oats, avenanthramides, help prevent free radicals from damaging LDL cholesterol, thus reducing the risk of cardiovascular disease. (*The Journal of Nutrition*, June 2004)

Oats are also a very good source of selenium. A necessary cofactor of the important antioxidant, glutathione peroxidase, selenium works with vitamin E. These powerful antioxidant actions make selenium helpful in decreasing asthma symptoms and in the prevention of heart disease. In addition, selenium is involved in DNA repair and is associated with a reduced risk for cancer, especially colon cancer.

Quinoa

Quinoa is high in complete protein, including all nine essential amino acids. Quinoa is especially high in the amino acid lysine, essential for tissue growth and repair.

Quinoa is a very good source of manganese as well as a good source of magnesium, iron, copper and phosphorous, this "grain" may be especially valuable for persons with migraine headaches, diabetes and atherosclerosis.

Magnesium helps relax blood vessels, preventing the constriction and rebound dilation characteristic of migraines. Increased intake of magnesium has been shown to be related to a reduced frequency of headache episodes. Magnesium's relaxing effect on blood vessels can also benefit blood pressure and heart health.

Quinoa is also a good source of riboflavin (vitamin B-2), which is necessary for proper cellular energy production. Riboflavin has been shown to help reduce the frequency of attacks in migraine sufferers, most likely by improving energy metabolism within brain and muscle cells.

SPICES & HERBS

Basil

The unique flavonoids (orientin and vicenin) found in basil protect at the cellular level. They protect cell structures as well as chromosomes from radiation and oxygen-based damage. In addition, basil provides protection against unwanted bacterial growth. These "anti-bacterial" properties of basil are not associated with its unique flavonoids, but instead with its volatile oils (estragole, linalool, cineole, eugenol, sabinene, myrcene, and limonene). Lab studies show the effectiveness of basil in restricting growth of numerous bacteria, including: Listeria monocytogenes, Staphylococcus aureus, Escherichia coli O:157:H7, Yersinia enterocolitica, and Pseudomonas aeruginosa.

Essential oil of basil, obtained from its leaves, has demonstrated the ability to inhibit several species of pathogenic bacteria that have become resistant to commonly used antibiotic.

Chili or Cayenne Peppers

These contain capsaicin, which makes them "hot". Topically, chilies relieve pain, as capsaicin stimulates certain nerve cells to release Substance P, which sends pain signals through-out the nervous system. Capsaicin quickly depletes the cells of substance P, thus temporarily blocking their ability to transmit pain impulses. Capsaicin ointments are commonly used to alleviate the pain of arthritis and shingles.

Taken internally, capsaicin triggers the release of endorphins in the brain, which has a pain-relieving effect similar to morphine.

Chills also speed up your metabolism (as much as 25%) which is why after eating hot peppers, you tend to sweat. As a thermogenic, hot peppers may even be an effective weight loss aid. Cayenne stimulates the production of gastric juices and helps relieve gas.

chilies can also help alleviate the symptoms of the common cold by breaking up congestion and keeping the airways clear. Chili peppers are also rich in beta-carotene and vitamin C. chilies may also help lower LDL cholesterol and triglycerides. They also contain antioxidant properties, which help protect against cancer and heart disease. Chili peppers can also prevent blood clots by extending blood coagulation time.

Cilantro/Coriander Seeds

Coriander's healing properties can be largely attributed to its exceptional phytonutrient content. Coriander's volatile oil is rich in beneficial phytonutrients, including carvone, geraniol, limonene, borneol, camphor, elemol, and linalool. Coriander's flavonoids include quercitin, kaempferol, rhamnetin, and epigenin. Plus, coriander contains active phenolic acid compounds, including caffeic and chlorogenic acid. Not only is coriander replete with a variety of phytonutrients, this exceptional herb emerged from our food ranking system as an important source of many traditional nutrients. Coriander is a good source of dietary fiber, iron, magnesium and manganese.

In Europe, coriander is referred to as an "anti-diabetic" plant. In parts of India, it is used for its anti-inflammatory properties. In the United States, coriander has recently been studied for its cholesterol-lowering effects.

Cinnamon

Cinnamon's unique healing abilities come from three basic types of components in the essential oils found in its bark. These oils contain cinnamaldehyde, cinnamyl acetate, and cinnamyl alcohol, plus a wide range of other volatile substances.

The cinnaldehyde in cinnamon helps prevent unwanted clumping of blood platelets. It inhibits the release of an inflammatory fatty acid called arachidonic acid from platelet membranes and reducing the formation of an inflammatory messaging molecule called thromboxane A2. Cinnamon's ability to lower the release of arachidonic acid from cell membranes also puts it in the category of an "anti-inflammatory" food that can be helpful in lessening inflammation.

Cinnamon's essential oils also qualify it as an "antimicrobial" food, and cinnamon has been studied for its ability to help stop the growth of bacteria as well as fungi, including the commonly problematic yeast Candida.

Cinnamon may significantly help people with type 2 diabetes improve their ability to respond to insulin, thus normalizing their blood sugar levels. Both test tube and animal studies have shown that compounds in cinnamon not only stimulate insulin receptors, but also inhibit an enzyme that inactivates them, thus significantly increasing cells' ability to use glucose.

Researchers from the US Agricultural Research

Service showed that less than half a teaspoon per day of cinnamon reduces blood sugar levels in persons with type 2 diabetes (not on insulin). Even the lowest amount of cinnamon, 1 gram per day (1/4 teaspoon), produced an approximately 20% drop in blood sugar; cholesterol and triglycerides were lowered as well. When daily cinnamon was stopped, blood sugar levels began to increase. (December 30, 2003)

Garlic *(See page 29)*

Ginger

Ginger, a common flavoring agent, has been used for thousands of years to treat numerous conditions including stomach aches, diarrhea, nausea, cholera, hemorrhaging, arthritis and toothaches.

In the U.S., ginger has been used primarily as a digestive aid and to help relieve excess gas and bloating; an aid in nausea, vomiting, morning sickness, and motion sickness; a diaphoretic (to induce sweating) and an appetite stimulant.

Ginger has a beneficial effect on our prostaglandins, and has shown to inhibits platelet aggregation (even more so than garlic or onions) and reduce inflammatory processes so is helpful for conditions such as arthritis, bursitis, tendonitis, injuries, and also allergies and asthma.

Rosemary

Rosemary, a commonly used flavoring agent, is finally getting the respect is deserves as a very powerful antioxidant. Rosemary contains Phytic acid, an anticarcinogenic polyphenol antioxidant component of dietary fiber that specifically affords possible protection against colorectal cancer. (Owen)

These natural polyphenols (carnosic acid) have also been studied for their inhibition potential for liver and lung cancers. (Offord)

Turmeric (Curry)

The primary spice in curry is turmeric which contains curcumin, the bright yellow pigment. Turmeric is a powerful medicine that has long been used in the Chinese and Indian systems of medicine as an anti-inflammatory agent to treat a wide variety of conditions, including flatulence, jaundice, menstrual difficulties, bloody urine, hemorrhage, toothache, bruises, chest pain, and colic.

Curcumin has been found to block activity of a hormone implicated in the development of colorectal cancer – results which contribute to a growing body of evidence pointing to the spice's cancer-fighting potential.

Researchers at the University of Texas Medical Branch at Galveston (UTMB) worked with curcumin and cell cultures to link a gastrointestinal hormone to the production of an inflammatory protein that accelerates the growth of a variety of cancer cells.

PHYTOCHEMICAL	HEALTH PROTECTIVE PROPERTY
Allylic sulfides	Inhibits cholesterol synthesis and protects against carcinogens
Alpha-linolenic acid	Reduces inflammation and stimulates the immune system
Carotenoids	Antioxidant that protects against cancer and may help reduce accumulation of arterial plaque
Catechins	Studies have linked catechins to low rates of gastrointestinal cancer; may aid the immune system and lower cholesterol
Coumarins	Prevents blood clotting and may have anti-cancer activity
Flavonoids	Block receptor sites for certain hormones involved in cancer promotion
Canima-glutamy-lallylic cysteines	May have a role in lowering blood pressure, and elevating immune system activities
Indoles	Induce protective enzymes that deactivate estrogen
Isothiniocyanates	Powerful inducers of protective enzymes
Limonoids	Powerful inducers of protective enzymes
Lycopene	Powerful carotenoid antioxidant that helps the body resist cancer and its progression
Monoterpenes	Cancer-fighting antioxidants that inhibit cholesterol production and aids protective enzyme activity
Phenolic acids	May help the body resist cancer by inhibiting nitrosamine formation and affecting enzymes
Phthalides	Stimulate the production of beneficial enzymes that detoxify carcinogens
Plant sterols	Block estrogen promotion of breast cancer activity, help block the absorption of cholesterol
Polyacetylenes	Protect against certain carcinogens found in tobacco smoke and help regulate prostaglandins
Triterpenoids	Prevents dental decay and acts as an anti-ulcer agent. Binds to estrogen and inhibits cancer by suppressing unwanted enzyme activity

FOUND IN FOODS SUCH AS:

Aged garlic extract

Flaxseed, soy products, purslane, walnuts

Parsley, carrots, winter squash, sweet potatoes, yams, cantaloupe, apricots, spinach, kale, turnip greens, citrus fruits

Green tea, berries

Parsley, carrots, citrus fruits

Parsley, carrots, citrus fruits, broccoli, cabbage, cucumbers, squash, yams, tomatoes, eggplant, peppers, soy products, berries

Aged garlic extract

Cabbage, Brussels sprouts, kale

Mustard, horseradish, radishes

Citrus fruits

Tomatoes, red grapefruit

Parsley, carrots, broccoli, cabbage, cucumbers, squash, yams, tomatoes, egg-plant, peppers, mint, basil, citrus fruits

Parsley, carrots, broccoli, cabbage, tomatoes, eggplant, peppers, citrus fruits, whole grains, berries

Parsley, carrots, celery

Broccoli, cabbage, cucumbers, squash, sweet potatoes yams, tomatoes, eggplant, peppers, soy products, whole grains

Parsley, carrots, celery

Citrus fruit:, licorice-root extract, soy products

Bibliography

Ames BN; Shigenaga MK; Hagen TM Oxidants, antioxidants, and the degenerative diseases of aging. Division of Biochemistry and Molecular Biology, University of California, Berkeley 94720. Proc Natl Acad Sci U S A 1993 Sep 1;90(17):7915-22

Aquino R; et al. New polyhydroxylated triterpenes from Uncaria tomentosa. J Nat Prod 1990 May-Jun;53(3):559-64

Aquino R; De Simone F; et al Plant metabolites. Structure and in vitro antiviral activity of quinovic acid glycosides from Uncaria tomentosa and Guettarda platypoda. J Nat Prod 1989 Jul-Aug;52(4):679-85

Asano Y; Okamura S; et al *Effect of (-)-epigallocatechin gallate on leukemic blast cells from patients with acute myeloblastic leukemia.* Life Sci 1997;60(2):135-42

Awasthi S; Srivatava SK; Piper JT; Singhal SS; Chaubey M; Awasthi YC Curcumin protects against 4-hydroxy-2-trans-nonenal-induced cataract formation in rat lenses. Am J Clin Nutr 1996 Nov;64(5):761-6

Barch DH; Rundhaugen LM Ellagic acid induces NAD(P)H:quinone reductase through activation of the antioxidant responsive element of the rat NAD(P)H:quinone reductase gene. Carcinogenesis 1994 Sep;15(9):2065-8

Block, Gladys, et al "Fruit, Vegetable and Cancer Protection: A Review of the Epidemiological Evidence," Nutrition and Cancer, 1992, Vol 17: 2, 1-29.

Byers, Tim, et al. "Dietary Carotenes, Vitamin C and Vitamin E as Protective Antioxidants in Human Cancers." Annual Rev. Nutrition, 1992, 12: 139-59.

Cao J; Xu Y; Chen J; Klaunig JE Chemopreventive effects of green and black tea on pulmonary and hepatic carcinogenesis. Fundam Appl Toxicol 1996 Feb;29(2):244-50

Cheshier JE; Ardestani-Kaboudanian S; et al Immunomodulation by pycnogenol in retrovirus-infected or ethanol-fed mice. Life Sci 1996;58(5):PL 87-96

Chopra, M. et al "Free Radical Scavenging of Lutein" Carotenoids in Human Health, Ann NY Acad Sci, 1993, Vol 691, 246-249.

Digiesi V; Cantini F; et al Coenzyme Q10 in essential hypertension. Mol Aspects Med 1994;15 Suppl:s257-63

Diplock AT Antioxidant nutrients and disease prevention: an overview. Am J Clin Nutr 1991 Jan;53(1 Suppl):189S-193S

Ding M; Wang S; Journal of Biological Chemistry , June 2006 (Vol. 281, Issue 25, 17359-17368).

Ellouali M; Boisson-Vidal C; Durand P; Jozefonvicz J Antitumor activity of low molecular weight fucans extracted from brown seaweed Ascophyllum nodosum. Anticancer Res 1993 Nov-Dec;13(6A):2011-9

Fokina GI; Roikhel' VM; Frolova MP; Frolova TV; Pogodina VV [The antiviral action of medicinal plant extracts in experimental tick-borne encephalitis] Vopr Virusol 1993 Jul-Aug;38(4):170-3

Grassel E *Effect of Ginkgo-biloba extract on mental performance. Double-blind study using computerized measurement conditions in patients with cerebral insufficiency* Fortschr Med 1992 Feb 20;110(5):73-6

Guo Q; Zhao B; Li M; Shen S; Xin W *Studies on protective mechanisms of four components of green tea polyphenols against lipid peroxidation in synaptosomes.* Biochim Biophys Acta 1996 Dec 13;1304(3):210-22

Harttig U; Hendricks JD; et al. Organ specific, protocol dependent modulation of 7,12-dimethyl-benz[a]anthracene carcinogenesis in rainbow trout (Oncorhynchus mykiss) by dietary ellagic acid. Carcinogenesis 1996 Nov;17(11):2403-9

Hollman PC; van Trijp JM; Mengelers MJ; de Vries JH; Katan MB Bioavailability of the dietary antioxidant flavonol quercetin in man. Cancer Lett 1997 Mar 19;114(1-2):139-40

Hocman G Prevention of cancer: vegetables and plants. Research Institute of Preventive Medicine, Bratislava, Czechoslovakia. Comp Biochem Physiol [B] 1989; 93(2):201-12

Hollman PC; et al, Absorption and disposition kinetics of the dietary antioxidant quercetin in man. Free Radic Biol Med 1996;21(5):703-7

Iizima-Mizui N; Fujihara M; Himeno J; Komiyama K; Umezawa I; Nagumo T Antitumor activity of polysaccharide fractions from the brown seaweed Sargassum kjellmanianum. Kitasato Arch Exp Med 1985 Sep;58(3):59-71

Itoh H; Noda H; Amano H; Zhuaug C; Mizuno T; Ito H Antitumor activity and immunological properties of marine algal polysaccharides, especially fucoidan, prepared from Sargassum thunbergii of Phaeophyceae. Anticancer Res 1993 Nov-Dec;13(6A):2045-52

Kamei H; Kojima T; Hasegawa M; Koide T; Umeda T; Yukawa T; Terabe K "Suppression of tumor cell growth by anthocyanins in vitro." Cancer Invest 1995; 13(6):590-4

Knekt P; Jarvinen R; Seppanen R; Rissanen A; and others Dietary antioxidants and the risk of lung cancer. Am J Epidemiol 1991 Sep 1;134(5):471-9

Kochi M; Isono N; et al Antitumor activity of a benzaldehyde derivative.Cancer Treat Rep 1985 May;69(5):533-7

Kuo ML; Huang TS; Lin JK Curcumin, an antioxidant and anti-tumor promoter, induces apoptosis in human leukemia cells. Biochim Biophys Acta 1996 Nov 15;1317(2):95-100

Laplaud PM; Lelubre A; Chapman MJ Antioxidant action of Vaccinium myrtillus extract on human low density lipoproteins in vitro: initial observations. Fundam Clin Pharmacol 1997;11(1):35-40

Muramatsu K; Fukuyo M; Hara Y Effect of green tea catechins on plasma cholesterol level in cholesterol-fed rats. J Nutr Sci Vitaminol (Tokyo) 1986 Dec;32(6):613-22

Nowicky JW; Staniszewski A; et al Evaluation of thiophosphoric acid alkaloid derivatives from Chelidonium majus L. ("Ukrain") as an immunostimulant in patients with various carcinomas. Drugs Exp Clin Res 1991;17(2):139-43

Offord EA; Mace K; Avanti O; Pfeifer AM Mechanisms involved in the chemoprotective effects of rosemary extract studied in human liver and bronchial cells. Nestle Research Centre, Lausanne, Switzerland. elizabeth. Cancer Lett 1997 Mar 19;114(1-2):275-81

Owen RW; Faecal phytic acid and its relation to other putative markers of risk for colorectal cancer. Gut 1996 Apr;38(4):591-7

Packer L, Witt EH, Tritschler HJ, Alpha-Lipoic acid as a biological antioxidant. Free Radic Biol Med 1995 Aug;19(2):227-50

Packer, L., "Protective role of Vitamin E in biological systems. Am J Clin Nutr 1991 Apr;53(4 Suppl):1050S-1055S.

Packer L., Suzuki, "Vitamin E and Alpha-Lipoate: Role in Antioxidant Recycling and Activation of the NF-KB Transcription Factor" Molec. Aspects med. (1993).

Palan, Prabhududas, "Antioxidant Vitamins & Cancer" The Nutrition Report Oct. 1991.

Pietri S; Maurelli E; Drieu K; Culcasi M *Cardioprotective and anti-oxidant effects of the terpenoid constituents of Ginkgo biloba extract (EGb 761).* J Mol Cell Cardiol 1997 Feb;29(2):733-42

Maitra I; Marcocci L; Droy-Lefaix MT; Packer L *Peroxyl radical scavenging activity of Ginkgo biloba extract EGb 761.* Biochem Pharmacol 1995 May 26;49(11):1649-55

Rai GS; Shovlin C; Wesnes KA A double-blind, placebo controlled study of Ginkgo biloba extract ('tanakan') in elderly outpatients with mild to moderate memory impairment. Curr Med Res Opin 1991;12(6):350-5

Rao, H. et al "Influence of Beta Carotene on Immune Function" Carotenoids in Human Health, Ann NY Acad Sci, 1993, Vol 691, 262-264.

Rice-Evans CA; et al The relative antioxidant activities of plant-derived polyphenolic flavonoids. Free Radic Res 1995 Apr;22(4):375-83

Rizzi R; Re F; Bianchi A; De Feo V; et al Mutagenic and antimutagenic activities of Uncaria tomentosa and its extracts. J Ethnopharmacol 1993 Jan;38(1):63-77

Rong Y; Li L; Shah V; Lau BH Pycnogenol protects vascular endothelial cells from t-butyl hydroperoxide induced oxidant injury. Biotechnol Ther 1994-95;5(3-4):117-26

Sagesaka-Mitane Y; Miwa M; Okada S Platelet aggregation inhibitors in hot water extract of green tea. Chem Pharm Bull (Tokyo) 1990 Mar;38(3):790-3

Senatore A; Cataldo A; Iaccarino FP; Elberti MG [Phytochemical and biological study of Uncaria tomentosa] Boll Soc Ital Biol Sper 1989 Jun;65(6):517-20

Sobota, A.E. Inhibition of Bacterial Adherence by Cranberry Juice: Potential use for the treatment of urinary tract infections. Journal of Urology (May 1884(131: 1013-16

Stoll S; Scheuer K; Pohl O; Muller WE *Ginkgo biloba extract (EGb 761) independently improves changes in passive avoidance learning and brain membrane fluidity in the aging mouse.* Pharmacopsychiatry 1996 Jul;29(4):144-9

Stoner GD; Mukhtar H Polyphenols as cancer chemopreventive agents. J Cell Biochem Suppl 1995;22:169-80

Taborska E; Bochorakova H; et al, [The greater celandine (Chelidonium majus L.)--review of present knowledge] Ceska Slov Farm 1995 Apr;44(2):71-5

Takehara, M. et al Isolation and anti-viral activities of the Double-strained RNA from Leninus Edodes (Shiitake). Kobe Journal of Mecial Science Aug. 1984, 30 (3-4):25-34.

Thomas SR; Neuzil J; Stocker R Cosupplementation with coenzyme Q prevents the prooxidant effect of alpha-tocopherol and increases the resistance of LDL to transition metal-dependent oxidation initiation. Arterioscler Thromb Vasc Biol 1996 May;16(5):687-96

Tixier JM; et al Evidence by in vivo and in vitro studies that binding of pycnogenols to elastin affects its rate of degradation by elastases. Biochem Pharmacol 1984 Dec 15;33(24):3933-9

Tsuda H; et al., Chemopreventive effects of beta carotene, alpha-tocopherol and five naturally occurring antioxidants on initiation of hepatocarcinogenesis by 2-amino-3-methylimidazo[4,5-f]quinoline. Jpn J Cancer Res 1994 Dec;85(12):1214-9

Wagner H; Kreutzkamp B; Jurcic K [The alkaloids of Uncaria tomentosa and their phagocytosis-stimulating action] Planta Med 1985 Oct;(5):419-23

Warot D; Lacomblez L; et al Comparative effects of ginkgo biloba extracts on psychomotor performances and memory in healthy subjects Therapie 1991 Jan-Feb;46(1):33-6

White HL; Scates PW; Cooper BR Extracts of Ginkgo biloba leaves inhibit monoamine oxidase. Life Sci 1996;58(16):1315-21

Xiaofu Wang et al. "Curcumin inhibits neurotensin-mediated interleukin-8 production and migration of HCT116 human colon cancer cells." Clinical Cancer Research. Sep 15, 2006; 12 (18).

Zhao BL; Li XJ; He RG; Cheng SJ; Xin WJ *Scavenging effect of extracts of green tea and natural antioxidants on active oxygen radicals.* Cell Biophys 1989 Apr;14(2):175-85

Zhuang C; Itoh H; Mizuno T; Ito H Antitumor active fucoidan from the brown seaweed, umitoranoo (Sargassum thunbergii). Biosci Biotechnol Biochem 1995 Apr;59(4):563-7

# of copies	TO PLACE AN ORDER:

___	*Aspirin Alternatives: The Top Natural Pain-Relieving Analgesics* (Lombardi)	$8.95
___	*Bilberry & Lutein: The Vision Enhancers!* (Ley)	$4.95
___	*Calcium: The Facts, Fossilized Coral* (Ley)	$4.95
___	*Castor Oil: Its Healing Properties* (Ley)	$3.95
___	*Dr. John Willard on Catalyst Altered Water* (Ley)	$3.95
___	*Chlorella: Ultimate Green Food (Ley)*	$4.95
___	*CoQ10: All-Around Nutrient for All-Around Health* (Ley)	$4.95
___	*Colostrum: Nature's Gift to the Immune System* (Ley)	$5.95
___	*DHA: The Magnificent Marine Oil* (Ley)	$6.95
___	*DHEA: Unlocking the Secrets/Fountain of Youth-2nd ed.* (Ash & Ley)	$14.95
___	*Diabetes to Wholeness* (Ley)	$9.95
___	*Discover the Beta Glucan Secret* (Ley)	$3.95
___	*Fading: One family's journey ... Alzheimer's* (Kraft)	$12.95
___	*Flax! Fabulous Flax!* (Ley)	$4.95
___	*Flax Lignans: Fifty Years to Harvest* (Sönju & Ley)	$4.95
___	*God Wants You Well* (Ley)	$14.95
___	*Health Benefits of Probiotics* (Dash)	$4.95
___	*How Did We Get So Fat? 2nd Edition* (Susser & Ley)	$8.95
___	*How to Fight Osteoporosis and Win!* (Ley)	$6.95
___	*Maca: Adaptogen and Hormone Balancer (Ley)*	$4.95
___	*Marvelous Memory Boosters* (Ley)	$3.95
___	*Medicinal Mushrooms: Agaricus Blazei Murill* (Ley)	$4.95
___	*MSM: On Our Way Back to Health W/ Sulfur* (Ley) SPANISH	$3.95
___	*MSM: On Our Way Back to Health W/ Sulfur* (Ley)	$4.95
___	*Natural Healing Handbook* (Ley)	$14.95
___	*Nature's Road to Recovery: Nutritional Supplements for the Alcoholic & Chemical Dependent* (Ley)	$5.95
___	*PhytoNutrients: Medicinal Nutrients in Foods- Revised /Updated* (Ley)	$5.95
___	*Recipes For Life! (Spiral Bound Cookbook)* (Ley)	$19.95
___	*Secrets the Oil Companies Don't Want You to Know* (LaPointe)	$10.00
___	*Spewed! How to Cast Out Lukewarm Christianity Through Fasting and a Fasted Lifestyle* (Ley)	$15.95
___	*The Potato Antioxidant: Alpha Lipoic Acid* (Ley)	$6.95
___	*Vinpocetine: Revitalize Your Brain w/ Periwinkle Extract!* (Ley)	$4.95

Book subtotal $ _____ + $5.00 shipping = $_____

Credit card orders please call toll free: 1-877-BOOKS11
For more info visit: www.blpublications.com